ADVANCE PRAISE FOR FOOD BULLYING

"*Food Bullying* is a much-needed critiq
guilt over food choices. Payn, international award-winning author,
exposes the multi-trillion-dollar marketing and misrepresentation
of food meant to make you question and stress out over grocery
store purchases. Food bullies beware: the public deserves better and
finally has a voice defending their food choices."

~ **Dr. David Samadi**, *Urologic Oncologist Expert*
& World Renowned Robotic Surgeon

"As a Registered Dietitian Nutritionist, I try to be the advocate and
voice of reason for my clients and consumers. From food shaming and
scare tactics to hit lists and dreadlines, the state of the plate is fraught
with confusion, chaos and clutter. *Food Bullying* engages and enables
readers to overcome their fear to make shopping, food preparation
and eating enjoyable endeavors rather than a battleground."

~ **Leslie Bonci**, MPH, RDN, CSSD, LDN
Kansas City Chiefs Sports Dietitian

"Food cuts to the core of our identity and is laden with powerful
emotional associations. In *Food Bullying*, Michele Payn cuts a clear
trail through the jungle of nonsensical claims that unscrupulous
food marketers make, using fear to tap into these emotions, about
the supposed health benefits of food fads in their greedy attempts
to build market share. This book will banish the nagging guilt
one might feel passing over $8/gallon organic milk in favor of the
much more affordable and equally healthy conventional brands,
and guide consumers to sane, guilt-free shopping. Give a copy to
your food-fear obsessed friends. They'll thank you for it."

~ **L. Val Giddings**, PhD, *Senior Fellow*
Information Technology & Innovation Foundation

"*Food Bullying* is an insightful book into the world of food marketing and peer pressures. It highlights how some in the food industry have created fear-based campaigns to benefit their own margins or market share. Perhaps even more importantly, it takes readers on a self-evaluating journey toward recognizing that many of us may be unknowingly participating in one of the various forms of food bullying. This realization could be a crucial step toward ending the consumer confusion that food bullying perpetuates. This is a great read for all those who want to better understand food and the psychology behind it."

~ **Clinton Monchuk**, *Executive Director*
Farm & Food Care Saskatchewan

"Michele Payn has consistently provided a calming voice in the conversation about food and farming. In her latest book, she takes on the very real problem of food bullying, how customers can recognize and deal with this behavior, and how professionals in nutrition and health can help counteract this negativity with facts and science."

~ **Leah McGrath** RDN, LDN
Founder of Buildup Dietitians, Retail Dietitian

"Something that should be one of the simple joys in life, nurturing ourselves and our families with food, has gotten so complicated— caught up in mistrust that is made worse by meaningless labels. Consumers just want to make the right choices, but they are too often confused and manipulated. The solution is facts, and that's what Michele Payn serves up in her latest book. By helping readers separate "bull speak" from facts, Payn is empowering informed consumer choice and a food system that truly will sustain us."

~ **Zippy Duvall**, *President*
American Farm Bureau Federation

"People are hungry for accurate, positive, and meaningful information that empowers them to enjoy their food with health in mind. This book helps people avoid the B.S. so they can make their own, well-informed decisions based on facts, not fear."

~ **Melissa Joy Dobbins,** MS, RDN, CDE
The Guilt-Free RD®

"In her third book, Michele Payn continues to connect personal stories and science. *Food Bullying* addresses the ongoing issue of the psychology of food marketing and guides consumers through the web of misinformation in food choices, diets, and eating decisions. In today's polarized food conversation about 'good' vs. 'bad', 'right' vs 'wrong' eating, this book helps people wade through the Bull Speak."

~ **Jennifer Schmidt**, *Registered Dietitian & Farmer*

Food Bullying

FOOD
BULLYING

How to Avoid Buying B.S.

MICHELE PAYN

NEW YORK

LONDON • NASHVILLE • MELBOURNE • VANCOUVER

FOOD BULLYING

How to Avoid Buying B.S.

Published in New York, New York, by Morgan James Publishing. Morgan James is a trademark of Morgan James, LLC. www.MorganJamesPublishing.com

ISBN 9781642794090 paperback
ISBN 9781642794106 eBook
Library of Congress Control Number: 2018914588

COVER PHOTOS: Food image provided by Emma Stoltzfus at PhotographBug.
Graphics in Chapters 1, 5, 12, 18 & 19 provided by Hannah Myers at Hannah Myers Creates.
Graphics in Chapters 10 & 16 provided by Icons made by Freepik from flaticon.com.

Cover Design by:
Rachel Lopez
www.r2cdesign.com

Interior Design by:
Chris Treccani
www.3dogcreative.net

Morgan James is a proud partner of Habitat for Humanity Peninsula and Greater Williamsburg. Partners in building since 2006.

Get involved today! Visit
MorganJamesPublishing.com/giving-back

DEDICATION

*To every person who has been shamed
about your food or farming choices:
may this book give you the courage
to stand up to the bullies.*

CONTENTS

INTRODUCTION

Are you buying B.S. (Bull Speak)?

Is non-GMO, gluten-free, antibiotic-free, fat-free milk better than regular milk?

Are "all-natural" corn chips better for you?

Does anyone really need organic, natural, hormone-free cat litter?

"No" should be the quick, simple answer to each of those questions. No to milk carrying too many label claims, no to all-natural corn chips, and, most certainly, no to kitty litter B.S. (Bull Speak) marketing claims. And no to the bullying that is clearly happening across dinner plates, grocery aisles, and food deliveries.

However, I recognize that saying "no" is difficult, just as it is on the playground. People feel judged and bullied around food. Hundreds of examples of food bullying poured in while I was writing this book. Friends, people on social media, and audience members were happy to share because every food experience has a story. What's yours? Is your food defined by image, what your friends tell you on Facebook, the brand on the bag, or the simple sensory pleasure food provides? How do others influence your food story? When and where do you need to say no?

xiv | FOOD BULLYING

Who doesn't love a good story? Whether it's reading a fairytale to a child and watching her eyes light up, spinning tales to entertain your friends over cocktails, the folklore found across family traditions, or losing yourself in a movie—we all enjoy stories. They make us feel good, provide us with connectivity, and drive our decisions.

Positioning one food as superior to another

Food, once cherished for nourishment, has become a chaotic playground filled with claims to bully and even demonize people around their eating choices. The need to position one food as superior to another lies at the heart of food bullying. Fat-free marshmallows. Gluten-free water. Grass-fed peaches. Hormone-free salt. Vegan water. No-salt added, boneless bananas. Somehow, our hunger for a feel-good story about our food has led to these ludicrous labels. I call B.S.!

Sixty percent of Americans say food labels influence their food purchases. Consider this scenario in your meat case or butcher shop. Company X decides to proclaim its chicken is "antibiotic-free." Suzie consumer is left to wonder what is wrong with the other chicken. Are there antibiotics in it?

"Am I doing the right thing for my family?" is Suzie's first question. As a mom, I completely understand that question—and ask myself that frequently. Instead, I suggest you start with "why are they making this claim?" I call this the "WHY? fear filter" and explain it in greater detail in Chapter 20.

If you don't pause to ask yourself about why there is marketing on labels, you have just been bullied by an inanimate object—in fact, the label itself. How? In the "antibiotic-free" meat case example above, there is nothing wrong with the other chicken; all meat goes through the same federally-mandated approval process to protect you from antibiotics.

However, company X's label claim infers superiority and creates fear about the other products. Remember, a company wants to differentiate its product so you spend money on its brand. Fear and suspicion are keys to bullying; both create a vicious cycle that leads to more B.S. food and behavior.

It's tiring. I've watched that bullying cycle continue in restaurants and across the grocery store, from meat to milk to eggs to produce to grains. It's time for food bullying to stop—and that starts with you not buying B.S. food.

Five ways to avoid buying B.S. food

I'll take a deeper dive into each of these throughout *Food Bullying*, but I wanted to give you a handful of quick tips because I know your time is valuable. I'll be covering each in further detail with examples throughout this book.

1. **Ignore empty food claims.** Just as you don't want food with empty calories, avoid food with empty label claims such as "____-free," "all-natural," "farm-raised," or "sustainable." For example, all milk in the grocery store is non-GMO, gluten-free, and antibiotic-free. Those labels are not measurable or meaningful but are used to make one product seem more attractive than another. If you want to know facts—not B.S., flip the package over, and read the Nutrition Facts Label, which is scientifically true.

2. **Understand the journey.** The journey of your food is an amazing story—and usually not the negative, sensationalized claims you saw on YouTube or Netflix. Sometimes, many hands are involved in producing your food. In other cases, such as a bag of apples, the last hand to touch the apple was the one that picked it from the tree. In every case, rules are in place for proper food handling to ensure it is safe and nutritious when it reaches your table.

Rather than buying B.S., get to know the rigorous system and science in place to protect your food safety.

3. **Stand up to the bullies.** Often a food claim is communicated in a way designed to create an extreme emotional response. People become scared; even well-intentioned neighbors and friends can pressure you to change your eating and buying habits. Celebrities, wellness gurus, or gym nutritionists often proclaim their way is the only right way. Who are they to say your food isn't good enough? Your family's nutrition is your business. Just as bullying is a real threat in our schools, food bullying is getting out of hand and takes advantage of insecurity. Make your food decisions based on science and find experts with firsthand experience to help you, such as a Registered Dietitian Nutritionist (RDN), food scientist, or farmer.

4. **Get to know the people.** Have you watched a documentary on farmers abusing animals, damaging the environment, or operating huge factory farms? In reality, 96% of today's U.S. farms and ranches are still run by families; they are the people who can give you the real story about how food is raised, without the B.S. Seven out of 10 Americans believe it's important to know the farmers who produce their food. And yet, in the earlier chicken meat case example, a common question is: "Why are farmers pumping antibiotics into chicken?" If you talk with a farmer, you'll find that it's often cruel to withhold medicine when chickens are sick and, even then, the dosage is strictly regulated by federal policies. That poultry farmer can also explain the many steps he takes, under federal requirement, to be sure all your chicken isn't chocked full of antibiotics—even the meat in the packages without an "antibiotic-free" label.

5. **Make your own decisions.** Have you felt pressured by groupthink? Define your own health, ethical, environmental, and social standards when it comes to food. And measure all claims against YOUR OWN standards rather than falling prey to B.S. claims and behaviors.

After a lifetime on a farm and, more recently, writing two books about food, I've come to realize that I am confident in my standards because of my firsthand understanding of the science, source, and system behind food. I hope to share enough of that with you to help you become as equally as clear about your own standards. Those standards and knowing your own food story, are your answer to bullying.

Why this book?

Many people will tell you a beautiful story about how food is raised on perfect farms by wonderful people, making you feel good about your eating choices. However, truth in food matters more to me than simply helping you feel good. It's more important to me that you understand where food comes from and how you've likely fallen for B.S. food in pursuit of a perfect story.

I see my friends confused, people questioning what has happened to food, and the bullying getting increasingly out of hand after 18 years of working to connect farm and food. I also know how the chaos around food has hurt family farms and want to do something to help people who are raising our food.

In short, the fascination for finding the "perfect" food story that makes the "right" social statement has led to an inability to discern B.S. from meaningful information. I wrote this book to equip you to find the signposts of food bullying, make more rational decisions, and avoid buying B.S. on the chaotic food playground.

Elevate the food conversation

Food is a basic necessity, not an opportunity for manipulation. It is time to elevate the food conversation above B.S. so you can avoid frustration and anxiety the next time you are making eating choices. Hopefully, *Food Bullying: How to Avoid Buying B.S.* will help you do just that!

The book is arranged to first frame food bullying, including an examination of different levels of bullying and then to offer familiar examples of bully figures in food fairy tales and folklore. The third section outlines the who, what, why, where, when, and how in understanding food bullying, including what it's doing to our brains. The fourth section includes food label descriptions—and how you should manage and evaluate those to avoid information overload. The book's final section offers specific tools to help you find your own solutions, including your personalized action plan to help you create a better food story.

If *Food Bullying* gives you pause and compels you to ask "Why is that claim on my food?" whenever you make eating choices, I'll consider my mission accomplished. Hopefully, exposing the food bullies and their manipulation will inspire you to have greater confidence in your food-related decisions and more civilized conversations about food and farming. Ultimately, that will lead to even greater food appreciation and enjoyment. After all, no one deserves B.S. in their food!

SECTION 1

Understanding the playground of food bullying

CHAPTER 1
What is B.S.?

D o you want irrefutable evidence? Most of us like concrete answers. Consider the popularity of genetic testing services and the technology using DNA to find family connections and prove our heritage. My friend Gina is a highly successful businesswoman, wife, mom, and grandma. She's a vibrant optimist and turned to Ancestry.com to identify her father after spending decades wondering about him.

"The science is now there, it can tell us definitely," notes Gina. She sent in what seemed like a giant cup of spit, entered her information in the database, and then waited. Nothing, aside from fifth cousins. Gina gave up. A year later, a woman contacted her through Facebook after finding Gina's name on the Ancestry site, which catalogs data from anyone who has had testing done. The site showed the two women were related more closely than first cousins. Upon chatting, they discovered they were sisters! Not only did Gina find her father, but also three other siblings to complete her family story. It wasn't a fairytale ending, but it was irrefutable proof.

What proof are you looking for to complete your food story? "The science is now there; it can

Bullying preys on fear created by B.S. claims about food.

tell us definitely." This is as true for food as it is for genetic testing; yet, we refuse to trust what we know as proof and allow the bullies to rule the food playground in hopes of finding a fairytale. This section is designed to explain the playground and how the chaos impacts our eating choices.

How have you been made to feel about food?

Has anyone ever made you feel bad about the food you choose to eat? Is it OK to shame people about their eating choices if it's not socially acceptable to shame people on race, religion, or sexual orientation? Why is a pregnant woman made to feel guilty if she's not buying the "right" label of food, or a new dad totally frustrated over the thousands of options found in the grocery store? Is it necessary for a college student to be shamed over her choice to eat meat or not?

B.S. refers to the bad behaviors, deceptive label claims, marketing half-truths, and other unnecessary drama surrounding our food plates today. Frankly, it's all just Bull Speak (B.S.). An $8 gallon of milk from a specialty store is not superior to a $2.99 gallon of milk from a convenience store. Both the perceived better label and resulting sense of superiority are often B.S. Assuming you are a better person because you bought the "right label" of food is no different than schoolyard bullying over the "right brand" of clothing.

Bullying operates from a point of privilege, preying on fear. Food marketing is often fear-based. This misleading marketing has made food overly emotional, to the point where our nutrition is seemingly trumped by moral statement. The resulting social movement has caused an alarming rise in food bullying. The more food bullying, the more B.S. food—and so the cycle continues.

Consider this; if the power in your food choices has shifted to what you read on marketing labels, you are likely being bullied. The front of food packages frequently contains misleading and

B.S. information—because companies want you to spend your money on their product. The Michigan State University (MSU) Food Literacy 2018 study showed that 87% of people are at least somewhat influenced by food labels in their food buying decisions. Do label claims influence your eating choices?

The Nutrition Facts Label, also known as the black and white box or "panel," contains the information you need to know. The Nutrition Facts Label was just updated after 20 years to better represent today's serving sizes, and will be covered in Chapter 16. You can find standardized serving size, calories, fat, protein, sodium, carbohydrates, added sugars, and other essential nutrition information in this box. All food must have the new label by 2021 and, because it is regulated, it's a label you can rely on.

Bullying is different than conflict

Merriam Webster defines bullying as "acts of written or spoken words intended to intimidate or harass a person." Bullying is a huge concern with young people today; I know from personal experience how painful it is, after being bullied as a seventh-grade girl in a new school system. Taunts from decades past are still a clear and painful memory.

The National Bullying Prevention Center clarifies the difference between bullying and conflict, which is a disagreement or argument in which both sides share their views. Conflict is an exchange, such as a debate about whether green or white grapes are better. Bullying is done with a goal to hurt, harm, or humiliate. It's often about having power and control over another. The power, real or otherwise, can include a group against an individual, one person being physically larger than another, or elevated social status. Bullies often perceive their targets as vulnerable in some way and find satisfaction in harming them.

In normal conflict, people self-monitor. They read cues when lines have been crossed and then modify behavior accordingly.

Those with empathy usually realize they have hurt someone and will want to stop negative behavior. Those intending to cause harm and whose behavior goes beyond normal conflict will continue their behavior, even when they know it's hurting someone, according to the National Bullying Prevention Center.

What does food bullying mean?

Bullying doesn't happen without fear—and there's a whole lot of fear in food today! Food bullying literally takes food out of someone's hand—by removing choice, creating emotion, or forcing an individual into groupthink mentality.

What does food bullying mean to you? It's likely different for everyone, but bullying typically appeals to esteem or belonging needs, which will be detailed in Chapter 9. It can be done with the best of intentions, or to change your buying behavior.

A California friend said "Food advice, while possibly meant well, is not welcome when delivered with an air of superiority." That scenario seems especially true with mothers snubbing other mothers because of their food choices. It's not the "right" brand on the bag, the label has the "wrong" claims, there is a "bad" ingredient, or the "right" certification is missing. The result is B.S. behavior. As Beth Moore said, the hardest thing about being a woman is often other women.

Dinosaur eggs and well-intended zealots

"I was at the self-checkout line with my son, and we were scanning items, when, all of a sudden, the employee in charge of that area rushed over to me and grabbed the box of oatmeal with dinosaur eggs out of my hands! She says to me, 'from one mom to another I have to tell you what I've heard. I heard there is Roundup in the dinosaur eggs in this oatmeal'," writes blogger Lisa Hauf.

"I think my mouth hit the floor at this point. I couldn't believe she grabbed the box of oatmeal from my hands. I was shocked. I must admit, I stumbled for words, trying to inform her of the facts I had recently read.

"The part that amazes me the most is this oatmeal is sold on the grocery store's shelves; yet, she felt a need to grab it out of my hands because it may be unsafe. I understand she meant well. She didn't want to see my family in any danger. I could tell she has a huge heart and only wanted the best for those around her. She was also incredibly kind when I suggested she read up on some of the facts about chemicals in our food, and I pointed her to the "On Your Table" blog. Before we judge others on their food purchases or even strip the food from their hand, let's be informed. Let's do our research."[1]

Amen, Lisa. Research matters—on all sides of the plate.

Having dinosaur eggs stripped from your hands in the grocery store shows how much insecurity there is about food today. I'm sure the grocery store employee didn't intend to bully Lisa. However, taking food from another is an act of bullying, as is removing choice, even when done with the best of intentions.

Food bullying levels

Food bullying levels vary from a zealot stripping a mom of cereal in the store to those who judge others' food choices to evangelizers dumping unsolicited information to those who taunt by embarrassing others to shaming to the full-fledged bully. Based on research and years of studying food conversations, I've outlined six general levels of bullying in the table below, which I'll describe throughout the remainder of Section 1.

FOOD BULLYING LEVELS

ZEALOT

Subscribing to one way as the "right" way. Any other way is wrong.

Example: My family will only eat organic. It is the only healthy food.

JUDGE

Judging others who do not make the same eating choices.

Example: Looks down their nose at another's school snack selection or grocery cart.

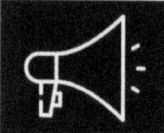

EVANGELIST

Giving unsolicited information to force your viewpoint on another.

Example: Animal rights activists on a college campus forcing grotesque pamphlets on a passerby or constantly posting your material on someone else's wall online.

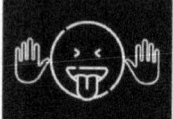

TAUNTER

Embarrassing others publicly to further your position, in person or online.

Example: Constantly questioning another person in your fitness class who makes different food choices.

SHAMER

Shaming others about their nutrition and food choice, publicly or privately.

Example: Insulting another parent in a mom group who cannot afford the preferred label or does not buy GMO-free.

BULLY

Bullying, which may include physical threats, attacks through social media, excluding from activities.

Example: Slandering a person on Facebook who stands for a way of eating, refusing to allow a certain parent to bring classroom treats because they're not made with "natural" ingredients, or vegans calling carnivores murderers.

Judging others on food

After zealots, like the dinosaur eggs bully, the next level looks at how you treat others about their food choices. Are you judging people if they make different eating choices? Several dietitians point to those who are yelling—and, consequently, judging—about a certain diet or ideology as the only correct way to eat, such as Paleo, Keto, low carb, high fat, and veganism. Judging happens across the spectrum.

Let me just pause to remind you—your eating choices are yours—and yours alone. You may be passionate about your way of eating, but can you guarantee it will work for someone else? Likely not. There are as many choices in how to eat as there are in what to eat—and no singular right answer.

As one bachelor friend pointed out, we are all guilty of food judgement, if we are honest. "I do that when someone is in the checkout line with me, holding on to a 12-pack of beer and a bag of chips." How many times have you considered others' grocery carts, judging their choices? Just do a gut check that your judgement doesn't turn into evangelizing, taunting, or shaming—or you, too, are a bully. We can all do better.

Taunting around the food plate

Bullying online has moved society to a new low, thanks to keyboard cowards. A small business owner recently shared a Facebook bullying episode. "I was called a murderer yesterday because I'm not vegan, and they said beef and dairy businesses were a 'horror show.' He also commented about my cat profile pic. I asked if I should have my cat arrested because he eats meat and must be a murderer, too." She then deleted the whole thread because she found it so upsetting.

On the flip side, not all vegans are rabid activists and some simply want to be free to make their own eating choices. If you're one of those people who have slipped meat into a vegan's dish as a joke, you're as guilty of taunting as the keyboard cowards above. Both are examples of food bullying. Let's respect choice, even when it's different than your own.

This also means we have to be more sensitive to those with food allergies. After explaining her severe food allergies, including the common allergy to peanuts, one woman shared her bullying experience. "I have had a co-worker place an open jar of peanuts on her desk every time that I was planning to meet with her in her office. The open peanuts meant I couldn't enter due to risk of severe reaction. Human resources staff and two of my superiors laughed it off saying they couldn't believe she would do that. Yet, she continued. It made work miserable." Taunting in a different form.

"I happily eat high fat, low carb and don't expect another soul to eat that way. It's my choice, and I don't need to be taunted by others," a mom in Texas summed it up perfectly.

Let's take a step back. Food is food. It's a basic necessity. Eating choices are personal. The food you choose to eat is personal. That is no reason for any level of bullying. There is irrefutable evidence about our eating choices, yet food continues to be highly emotional on the chaotic playground described in the next chapter.

Food shaming

As humans, we are driven towards social acceptance, and being excluded leads to fear. For example, a mom group determines it is necessary to purchase only organic products to be a "good" mom. Any mom not conforming to the "groupthink" will be questioned, shamed and then bullied into providing "acceptable" food or face social exclusion. Food shaming has become increasingly common in parenting groups; it's important to recognize that exclusion, social manipulation, and humiliation are all signs of bullying on the playground.

Creating doubt through marketing is another bullying behavior that encourages groupthink. This technique is seen in absence claims on food, claims such as hormone-free chicken. Imagine Chris, the consumer, in the grocery store, trying to quickly grab some chicken for dinner after a hectic day at work. "This package says no hormones. I saw on Facebook that chickens have bigger breasts because of hormones." A quick moment of confusion follows and doubt sets in. "Yikes, hormones can't be good. I'd better buy the package that says no hormones even if it costs more."

How is this bullying and B.S.? There are hormones in all food, unless you're having salt for a meal. Vegetables, maple syrup, and meat have hormones, just like every other piece of food on your fork. There are no hormones on the market to give to chickens. None. They have been illegal since the 1950s. Hormones have not made Dolly Parton chickens; they have larger breasts because that's what consumers have demanded. In other words, farmers have bred chickens with larger breasts because of eating choices. Marketing and groupthink tell you otherwise, but do not fall for hormone claims on poultry or you are being bullied.

Shaming around food is very real and increasingly common. One young mom told me, "My mom even did it to me without knowing it. I had to point it out to her; she didn't mean anything bad by it but made me feel bad for feeding my kids fruit snacks." Bullying can be done without words. "Food bullying means others shaming me, even with their eyes, over my personal food choices. Some of us are just doing the best we can," said another parent in a wealthy suburb.

"Somebody telling me I'm buying/eating incorrectly if I don't eat vegan or organic" is how a Wisconsin millennial summed up food bullying, while another local friend said, "It's simply someone belittling my eating choices without knowing the reason behind them." A Canadian baby boomer dad pointed to food evangelists who try to force their viewpoint on him.

You can't have that!

The playground of food bullying is crowded and includes different levels of bullies. The first step in avoiding B.S. food is to acknowledge the bad behaviors, misleading or false label claims, marketing half-truths, and other unnecessary drama on the playground of food bullying. All of these bullying behaviors have resulted in a "you can't have that" mentality because of food bullies. Next we'll look who is affected by bullying.

CHAPTER 2

Who are the victims?

Fat. You can't have that! What if sizzling meat from the grill, creamy cheeses, refreshing whole milk, and crispy bacon belong in a healthy diet, in spite of dire warnings about dietary fat? Investigative journalist Nina Teicholz went on a nine-year-long quest to show how the misinformation about dietary fat took hold in the scientific community and public imagination. Teicholz went against the grain by standing up for fat, authoring the best-selling book *The Big Fat Surprise*.

It's an interesting example of how we can all fall victim to bullying through groupthink, which I'll cover in this chapter. Teicholz explains why the Mediterranean Diet is not the healthiest, in spite of the popularity of low-fat in the nutrition community. She points to science showing that we have been needlessly avoiding meat, cheese, butter, and other fats.

Whether feeling guilty about fat, being told your restaurant food choice is "wrong," or the pressure you feel from an overly opinionated work colleague to

Food bullying victims span all levels of income and generations, pushing groupthink instead of personal choice.

make the "right" eating choice at dinner, food bullying impacts all of us negatively.

Bullying: emotional, social, verbal, and cyber

Exclusion, social manipulation, humiliation, and rumor mongering are all examples of emotional or social bullying. For example, the co-worker who decides you should not be in charge of snacks for your team anymore because you don't bring the "right" labels. Or the one who snubs you for going on a pre-packaged meal plan to lose weight?

On a larger, corporate scale, I would also describe many B.S. label claims, such as all-natural, sustainable, and farm-raised as emotional or social bullying on the food playground. Stay tuned for more on the neuroscience of this marketing ploy in Section 3.

Verbal bullying is easier to identify; it includes spreading rumors, making jokes about someone's difference, teasing, name calling, intimidating, threatening, and slandering. The most egregious example are animal rights activists who are known for threatening farmers and even breaking into their farms and damaging personal property. Activists publicly slander the farm families for raising food, calling them names such as murderers and rapists. These disgusting bullying tactics are extremely hurtful to the families involved who consider it a privilege to take care of animals so they can provide us with food.

The National Bullying Prevention Center describes cyberbullying well. "The internet has become the new bathroom wall. Cyberbullying is when the internet, cell phones or other devices are used to send or post text or images intended to hurt or embarrass another person." Examples include threats online, hate speech, ridiculing someone publicly in online forums, threats and posting lies, rumors, or gossip about the target, and encouraging others to distribute that information.[2]

Evangelizing online

I saw this firsthand several years ago when the Humane Society of the United States (HSUS) decided to send an email blast, encouraging people to post negative comments during an online Twitter discussion amongst ag folks, known as AgChat. We were having a conversation about animal welfare that night, and HSUS tried to cyberbully to gain attention by using an established platform of an existing Twitter chat. The community behind AgChat rallied and was able to keep the conversation positive and away from the HSUS evangelizers who were tweeting to condemn farmers and ranchers.

Sending harassing, embarrassing, or otherwise unwelcome text messages is another example of cyberbullying. Leah McGrath, a registered dietitian nutritionist (RDN) for a well-known grocery chain in the East, actually had the activist group Organic Consumers Association target her with a form letter sent to retailers. They sent hundreds of emails until her IT department set up blocks, and she continued receiving form emails for weeks. She chose to flip the narrative, called them out for bullying on social media, and forwarded the emails back to the Organic Consumers Association for months until the bad behavior stopped.

How do activists evangelize, taunt, shame, and bully?

"Over the past decade, they've done a lot of research to test which methods of advocacy work, and how and why people become vegetarians," writes Kelsey Piper. It turns out that it's pretty tough to convince people to become vegetarian, but not so hard to bully them into feeling bad about eating meat.

"Studies have looked into the effects of different persuasion efforts: leafletting, online ads, undercover investigations of farms, street protests. What they have found, for the most part, is that none of the things advocacy groups were doing had detectable effects—partially because of constraints on the research, and partially because the underlying effects seem to be small and hard to measure (if there were effects at all). The results, and what they mean, are still being hotly contested within the animal rights community. That disagreement underscores the steep challenge the animal rights community faces in trying to convince the rest of the world to give up meat.

"It also stands in sharp contrast to the repeated successes the advocacy movement has had in pursuing a different course: pressure campaigns against corporations. Advocates have convinced companies like Starbucks and General Mills, for instance, to source eggs for their products from cage-free farms through a mix of behind-the-scenes negotiation and protests."[3]

Eggs from chickens not raised in cages are not necessarily superior. The eggs section of my last book discusses Henny Penny, the laying hen, as well as studies showing that there is no single right answer to hen housing. "Isn't it more natural for Henny to be outside, pecking corn off the ground? It's also more natural for her to freeze to death, eat trash, be killed by predators, and poop on her egg (increasing your risk for salmonella). And if Henny Penny gets mad or her fellow chicken is ill, she may decide to peck the other chickens to death.

"As a result, most chickens live in a temperature-controlled barn in some sort of cage. The eggs immediately leave the cage so there is little exposure to bacteria from manure. Today's hens have constant access to food and water 24 hours a day, oblivious to the drama that surrounds them about housing. Critically thinking about housing instead of marketing labels would increase logic in the egg case and decrease food drama." In other words, chickens aren't the victims here, but you might be with these B.S. claims.

Where are nutrition experts on the playground?

Turning to experts is one of the best ways to kick drama off the playground. Those with the education and/or firsthand experience with raising food, the science of nutrition, and food safety can reduce your confusion about food and, consequently, the fear of food that bullies prey on. The challenge is that experts are sometimes targeted by activists.

Registered dietitian nutritionists (RDNs) spend years in school learning about the science of nutrition and are expected to make science-based recommendations, according to the Academy of Nutrition and Dietetics (AND). However, there is some question about what research dietetic and health college students are being fed today—particularly on the most contentious issues.

The chairperson of the Department of Food Science and Human Nutrition at Iowa State University, in a 2018 study about how health/dietetic college students are being educated about genetically modified organisms (GMOs), found:

1. Anti-GMO propaganda documentary films have become a prime source of misinformation.
2. Most dietetic teachers have no background in farming or health issues, but readily pass along anti-biotechnology propaganda as facts.
3. Scientists are frustrated trying to counter this tsunami of fear-mongering when colleges and universities promote the anti-GMO agenda.[4]

It concerns me that one-sided documentaries are being used by academia teaching dietitians who need a well-rounded viewpoint and are expected to make science-based recommendations around food. (Be sure to read Danielle's story in Chapter 19.) Biased education is a type of food bullying since it does not paint the complete picture of how food is produced, doesn't include farmers' expertise in food production, lacks facts, and incorporates propaganda/activist pressure into curricula instead of science.

Misinformation leads to far-reaching consequences

Whether you love or hate GMOs, this type of bias showcases the lack of science-based information about how food is raised. Inaccuracy and imbalanced information are the common denominators across the entire spectrum of food bullying. Consequences are far-reaching.

- **Food waste**: 40% of food is wasted in the U.S. Apples and potatoes, modified to eliminate browning, have the potential to significantly reduce food thrown out. Yet, both were immediately rejected by McDonalds and other restaurants because of concerns around consumer backlash.

- **Food costs:** Consumer food costs are increased by marketing moves and activist pressure that result in more regulation. For example, each family in Canada is expected to pay $400 more for groceries in 2019 as compared to 2018.[5] The price of food in the States has risen 26.8% over the last 10 years.[6]

- **Farmer mental health crisis:** Farmer suicide rates have increased dramatically and gained national recognition in both the U.S. and Canada. Much of the farm mental health crisis is due to the economic hardships and inability to continue farming. For many farmers, "being a farmer" defines who they are, and when they can no longer afford to farm, it is emotionally excruciating.

Food bullies pressure brands

Have you considered that your favorite brands have also been bullied? Rather than relying on experts who are involved in producing food or scientific proof about what is best for the animals, environment, or consumers, companies are increasingly being publicly pressured by activists.

"The most cost-effective way to help animals on factory farms seems to be campaigns targeting suppliers, not targeting consumers."[3] Before we go on, let's pause. What is a factory farm? It's hard to define and a degrading term to the families who grow your food. Families still own 96% of farms and ranches in the U.S., with comparable percentages in Canada. Take a moment to consider how degrading terms like "factory farms" are to these family farmers. These terms are an example of both verbal and emotional bullying, often started by activists.

Groupthink = victims

The victims of food bullying span all income levels and generations, individually and corporately. The effects of group thinking are far-reaching on a chaotic playground of food bullying. The next chapter details this playground and revisits the levels of bullying.

CHAPTER 3

Do we really need a $5.75 trillion playground?

Imagine a $5.75 trillion playground with 40,000 pieces of equipment. Wouldn't it be overwhelmingly grandiose and likely more than you could comprehend? What would your elaborate playground include? Mine would likely have a jetted tub, pretty dairy cattle, a chocolate fountain, a basketball hoop, spin bikes, great music, a beach with crashing waves, and a few other frivolous items. And a huge sign "No B.S. allowed."

Consider this; food is a $5.75 trillion industry. It is huge business; it includes grocery stores, restaurants, online food retailers, foods sold at convenience stores, food trucks, and more.[7] It's a playground ripe for bullying, particularly in the grocery store, where there are nearly 40,000 products on average.

Who can possibly comprehend 40,000 items in a single store? That's the same capacity as many professional baseball stadiums in the U.S. Overwhelming, to say the least—and an opportunity for food bullies to run amok and promote B.S. groupthink.

Chaos rules on the playground, creating confusion with overwhelming food claims.

21

Now consider each of the 40,000 items in a grocery store. If there are five claims on each product, that adds up to 200,000 marketing messages at a minimum. For example, you may have seen multiple options in the egg cases, including natural, antibiotic-free, GMO-free, grass-fed, omega-enhanced, and free range labels. How is someone supposed to sort through 200,000 messages when he goes into a grocery store?

Marketing capitalizes on fear

No wonder I feel bombarded while food shopping. Do you? The overwhelm leads to confusion. Confusion turns into fear, which empowers bullying. Marketing capitalizes on the fear, with food buyers as the victims of constant B.S. about the "right" food. Turn on the television, drive by a digital billboard, take a peek at Instagram, walk into any restaurant, or open up your weather app; food and drink marketing messages infiltrate our lives.

With all the ways people are modifying the way they eat, I hear 'food snarkiness' just about anywhere I go where food is served. What food snarkiness have you seen? The sheer number of products and choices in a grocery store makes it a playground for your brain to do somersaults in overload mode.

School activities aren't even immune. Most parents worry about their kids being bullied, but they may need to check their own behavior around food. As one mom told my friend Jennie, "I only bring organic fruit, and you always bring those fruit snacks, so don't sign up for the classroom snacks. You like to bring Capri Suns, so you can't be in charge of drinks either. Don't bring homemade cookies because you didn't use 'natural ingredients.'" Is that acceptable behavior?

In some cases, it gets worse with teachers shaming children about snacks, even in a public school in a middle-class community in northern Michigan. "Our kids are allowed to bring a midmorning snack to school. There have been many days when our daughter has been in tears with anxiety about what the teacher will say. She has been scolded for bringing in sugar-free Jell-O with fruit because the teacher thought it was a dessert. But they will allow her to bring in a whole box of Cheez-Its and eat as much as she'd like. That's not OK in our book.

"We've had conversations with the school about this, but have gotten nowhere. We pack baby carrots, apple slices, grapes, or other healthy choices because our first priority is to raise our daughter with a healthy relationship with food, not one where her food choice gives her anxiety because of the teacher's attitude towards food. The peer pressure for a nine-year-old girl around food is real," reports a frustrated dad.

Chaos rules the playground

The playground is chaotic. It reminds me of my first time navigating the Cairo airport alone; my senses were assaulted with vendors shouting in different languages, the frenzy of unknown procedures, security guards with machete guns, and unfamiliar smells. While I loved working with Egyptians for over a month, my solo airport experience was discomforting. The more my senses were assaulted, the less time for thinking. The less time for thinking, the more confusion and fear—two behaviors sought out by bullies.

The more noise on food, the less time for thinking, and the more likely you are to believe marketing misinformation. This might be Cheesecake Factory and the glutinous servings spread across an overwhelming menu, but their cheesecake reels people in. Some say farmers' markets and food co-ops are chaotic. You choose your chaos, but it seems present in everyone's life. Just know food chaos sets the stage for bullying.

RDN Cara Harbstreet describes food chaos as "the cycle of restrict-binge-shame that drives the diet industry." Take a look at the nearly $50 billion in supplement sales and $64 billion weight loss industry if you want to know how big the problem is. There is profit in chaos.

Bullying even extends to the gym. I frequently hear food bullying stories like, "If you don't buy the premium water bottle brands or fancy snacks, there are some who turn up their noses." Or of a "gym nutritionist" pushing products with all the health claims at the gym, adding to the confusion.

Many farmers consider the 815 million people who suffer chronic malnourishment as casualties of food chaos. That's one in every ten people who don't have adequate nutrition. Meanwhile, 40% of food in the U.S. is wasted, and developing countries are prevented from getting food because of political agendas.

Keyboard cowards and cyberbullying

Food bullying is most prevalent in social media. "The rise of the internet and other technology has led to a new, very serious form of bullying: cyberbullying. Cyberbullying is when the internet, cell phones or other devices are used to send or post text or images intended to hurt or embarrass another person," according to the National Bullying Prevention Center.

A key question: have social media bullies created the chaos? Or, has the chaos created bigger bullies on social media? The people quick to slam others who don't agree with their eating choice, those who threaten people with a different viewpoint and the like. I refer to them as "keyboard cowards." The legal definition of cyberbullying is "the verbal bullying of someone through the use of often anonymous electronic communication, such as online posts or text messages." (Merriam Webster)

Keyboard cowards refuse to stop when their position has been stated. Instead, flagrant insults, often of a personal nature, begin. I've had my integrity questioned, been threatened, and labeled as a "shill" since venturing into the social media arena in 2008— particularly when my viewpoints fly in the face of activists who represent million dollar organizations. It's taught me to have social media policies in place to protect me and others from the bullies.

Ridiculing someone publicly in online forums is an example of cyberbullying, as are threats, posting lies/rumors/gossip about the targeted person, or sending harassing messages. When was the last time you saw hate speech about politics, food, or race on social media? Again, that's bullying—and it's time to stand up to it. YOU are a key part of stopping it.

Media adds to the chaos

Regardless of how you describe it, chaos reigns supreme on today's food playground. Bullies disguised as media are on all corners of the playground, creating more chaos for the overfed and underfed, wealthy and poor, educated and uneducated. New bullies rise out of the chaos, adding yet more confusion and Bull Speak.

"Food articles in magazines and newspapers create chaos. Even if they don't think they're bullying, they're touting a certain kind of food that's often the most expensive," points out a communications expert. Another food scientist with four children refers to parenting magazines' coverage of food and nutrition. "Confused. Guilted. Shamed. Bullied. It's no wonder people end up in the two extremes in food choices."

Different levels of bullies on the playground

What happens when new information about food comes into your world? Do you look around the playground, trying to find clarity in the chaos? Take another look at the food bullying table. Which of the six levels of bullying do you fall into? What about the groups influencing you're eating choices? Consider these levels and then we'll address how food bullying affects us in the next chapter.

FOOD BULLYING LEVELS

ZEALOT

Subscribing to one way as the "right" way. Any other way is wrong.

Example: My family will only eat organic. It is the only healthy food.

JUDGE

Judging others who do not make the same eating choices.

Example: Looks down their nose at another's school snack selection or grocery cart.

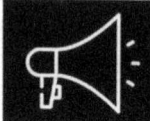

EVANGELIST

Giving unsolicited information to force your viewpoint on another.

Example: Animal rights activists on a college campus forcing grotesque pamphlets on a passerby or constantly posting your material on someone else's wall online.

TAUNTER

Embarrassing others publicly to further your position, in person or online.

Example: Constantly questioning another person in your fitness class who makes different food choices.

SHAMER

Shaming others about their nutrition and food choice, publicly or privately.

Example: Insulting another parent in a mom group who cannot afford the preferred label or does not buy GMO-free.

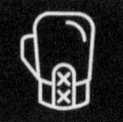

BULLY

Bullying, which may include physical threats, attacks through social media, excluding from activities.

Example: Slandering a person on Facebook who stands for a way of eating, refusing to allow a certain parent to bring classroom treats because they're not made with "natural" ingredients, or vegans calling carnivores murderers.

CHAPTER 4

How does food bullying affect us?

A bottle of hot dog water for $28. Found at a festival in Vancouver, Canada, the water with a floating weenie racked up $1,500 in sales. It was marketed as a miracle which "can help you look younger, reduce inflammation, and increase your brain function." It was also "keto-compatible and gluten-free."

Really.

Weenie water and psychology

"Hot dog water, in its absurdity, hopes to encourage critical thinking related to product marketing and the significant role it can play in our purchasing choices," said Douglas Bevans, the Hot Dog Water CEO.

It's an interesting look at the need to critically think about the food you're buying—or not buying. Hot dog water, along

Bullying creates confusion, guilt, distrust, higher priced food, a growing disconnect from the farm, and overall stress.

with its complementary products of breath spray, lip balm, and body fragrance, was a study in human behavior

"*Global News* reported that Bevans is actually a tour operator and an artist, and he created Hot Dog Water as a commentary on the "snake oil salesmen" of health and wellness marketing. *Psychology Today* cites a study published in the *Journal of Consumer Research* that calls this phenomenon affective conditioning, which is a transfer of feelings from one set of items to another."[8]

Fear trumps truth in food

I'll write more about the psychology of affective conditioning in later chapters, but this neuromarketing is a subtle bullying technique to influence our brains' emotional decisions while making food choices.

As a result of psychological maneuvering like this, the trust around food degrades, and the conversation often turns highly emotional. "Fear based marketing. Clouded with confusion. Fear trumps reason. Noisy minority agitates. Amazing technology misunderstood. Best intentions misconstrued." These are the typical descriptors offered by my Twitter community when asked to describe the climate around food.

"Food is safe, nutritious and wholesome," says Jennifer Schmidt, a dietitian and farmer in Maryland. "The climate around food is fear and falsehoods—a food fight." She's right. Little did I know when I wrote *No More Food Fights!* in 2013 that people would be buying weenie water five years later. Simply put, the side effects of food bullying are far-reaching, and the continued growth in food bullying has reached a point of needing national attention.

An obsession with healthy food

Have you heard of orthorexia? It's an obsession with eating foods one considers healthy. A person who suffers from this medical and psychological condition avoids specific foods in the belief that they are harmful. Even though people are eating healthy foods, it has detrimental health effects because of the limited food selection.

Social media posts and photos about meal preparation, including arrays of fruits and vegetables in colorful presentations, may increase orthorexia and malnutrition, according to nutrition experts and people who have experienced the eating disorder. RDN Christy Harrison says these images may convince people that is the right way to eat, but "we can't live off fruits and vegetables alone."[9]

Negative eating emotions have consequences

What if we enjoyed food instead of guilting others about eating choices and destroying relationships because of differences of opinion around nutrition? One of the dietary directives in Japan is to "enjoy your meals."

"There is a slew of evidence that eating-related pleasure, satisfaction, and enjoyment are important components of a healthy diet. At the same time, negative emotions related to eating like guilt, fear, shame, and judgment have real consequences for our health and well-being—and not just for social reasons."[10]

As I extensively wrote about in *Food Truths from Farm to Table*, food should be about celebration, nourishment, and family tradition. There's a downside to making people feel guilty, confused, and fearful of food—it shows up in your health and well-being. Keep that in mind as you make food selections.

Enjoying food is good for your health

To paraphrase dietitian Alissa Rumsey, this is what happens when you enjoy the food you eat:

1. *You'll digest your food better.* Enjoyment tells the parasympathetic nervous system to trigger its relaxation response. This is the same system that gets your digestion

going by relaxing the muscles in your gastrointestinal tract and increasing digestive juices.

2. *You'll absorb more nutrients.* When it comes to nutrient absorption, taste matters. A study looked at iron absorption when people from Sweden were given Thai food and people from Thailand were given Swedish food. In both cases, people absorbed less iron than when they ate the food from their native country, which they presumably enjoyed more.

3. *You'll be satisfied with less.* There is a difference between feeling physically full and feeling satisfied. If you aren't completely satisfied with the food you are eating, it becomes much easier to overeat.

Parental lunch competitions

Think back to when you were in school. Wasn't lunchtime a lot simpler? My ever-frugal mom put the simplest things she could in a paper bag, and I was happy to not eat school lunches, except for days when the cafeteria served tater tots. But today school lunch has become parental competition of who can make the cutest lunch packages with the best labels, coolest and most nutritious food that will make a social statement.

"There are two types of moms in this world when it comes to lunches, or so you think," blogger Nikki Pennington points out. "Moms who make lunches from scratch every single day with cookie cutters and love notes with freshly squeezed lemonade made with pure love. Then there are other moms, the moms like me, who hand pick Lunchables, lovingly peel off the wrapper of the said Lunchable, rearrange the crackers to make a nice little sandwich and write I love you with a permanent marker on the store-bought juice."

As Pennington goes on to explain, we don't always know the back story. She grew up with a single mom who couldn't afford things like Lunchables, and her mom usually didn't have time to make something homemade. "She was the mom who was working two jobs to make ends meet and putting herself through college at night. She was the mom who put me on the free lunch list at school because that's the only way I could get lunch. She was a really good mom regardless of whether my lunch was cookie cutter sandwich or a cheese spread with freshly squeezed drinks or perfect vegetables cut up from our garden."

Parental lunch competitions illustrate food shaming, but don't take into account the different lifestyles and struggles each family faces. What if money is tight, a parent (or child) has a disability that makes handcrafted bento boxes impossible, or a kid has a sensory disorder that limits his or her eating choice day after day? There are a variety of reasons why children might end up with the lunch they're eating on any given day. And wasting time judging each other over the contents of a lunchbox—or worse, shaming kids for what they eat at school—is pointless and hurtful.[11]

Why not celebrate the parent who does the cute cookie cutter sandwiches? And the parent who buys the pre-packaged meals, as well as the parent who buys a school lunch? They're all doing the best they can, and the end result is that kids are getting fed. Food should be about nourishment, not competition.

The playground is chaotic, but food doesn't need to be

Google brings up five million results for "understanding food labels." Chapters 15 and 16 will help outline the B.S. claims, and discuss in detail meaningful and measurable labels. There is no easy answer, particularly given all the players involved in food bullying—but I do suggest truth simplifies food. Confusion, guilt, distrust, higher priced food, malnourishment, a growing disconnect from the farm, and overall stress are just a few of the side effects of bullying.

Isn't it time we stand up for truth in food? My hope is that exposing bullies, their methods and motivators, along with providing examples of B.S. will help you navigate the playground and be on the lookout for food bullying.

In the next section, we will explore how fairytales filled with common food folklore abound across the playground.

SECTION 2

Recognizing food fairytales & folklore

CHAPTER 5

Can you find the wolf or ugly duckling?

B eautiful shoes at great prices. I love fun shoes, particularly when there's a story I can share with my friends and feel good every time I look at my new kicks. Apparently, I'm not the only one who likes a good shoe story, as Payless Shoes proved in Santa Monica in November 2018.

Under the name of "Palessi," the chain took over a former Armani store and filled it with $19.99 pumps and $39.99 boots. They then invited influencers to the grand opening of "Palessi" to get their opinions of the "designer" shoes.

"Party goers, having no idea they were looking at discount staples from the mall scene, said they'd pay hundreds of dollars for the stylish shoes, praising the look, materials, and workmanship. The top offer was $640, a mere 1,800% markup. Palessi sold about $3,000 worth of product in the first few hours of the stunt."[12]

It's amusing to think of shoe divas falling for shoes marked up 1,800% from bargain brands they likely would never consider. Same product, with a different story.

Food claiming "free-from" is Bull Speak (B.S.) and is not a healthier eating choice.

How does Palessi relate to grocery stores? Is one brand really superior or just a better story teller? Unfortunately, stories like "Palessi" are abundant in food, but less easily recognizable in a population that is three to four generations removed from a farm.

Fairytales are spun across the playground of food bullying, from the wicked wolf disguised as Little Red Riding Hood's grandma to taunts from Cinderella's stepsisters to Sleeping Beauty being bullied by the wicked fairy. All are levels of bullying, though the fairytales around food are not as well-known as our childhood folklore.

Stories seem to turn from reality to folklore the more removed people are from a place, product, or practice. The same is true in food; we live in a time when people are so hungry for the story behind their food that they often fall for folklore. Perhaps it's because so many feel more removed from how food is raised; some studies show that 75% of Americans haven't visited a farm in the last five years. It's hard to understand or trust what you don't know.

An absence of truth in food

This disconnect creates a need for quick-fix stories to make people feel good about food. My least favorite food folklore is known as absence-claim labeling, which infers superiority. Examples include hormone-free, gluten-free, HFCS-free, antibiotic-free, non-GMO, and preservative-free. Each of these claims is definitely not free from B.S.; yet 54% of consumers are looking for statements about the absence of certain ingredients.[13]

Consider the boy who cried wolf. He was a bored young boy sitting on the hillside watching the village sheep. He decided to amuse himself by crying out "Wolf, wolf…the wolf is chasing the sheep." The villagers came running, only to find the boy laughing in their faces. Of course, the villagers were angry, but the boy did it again—in spite of being warned not to cry wolf unless there was an actual emergency.

Later, the boy found a real wolf amongst his flock. He yelled wolf again and again, as loud as he could, but no one came running. When he didn't return to the village at sunset, everyone wondered where the boy was and went to find him. They found him crying on the hillside, the sheep scattered. An old man counseled him on the walk back to the village.

"Nobody believes a liar, even when he is telling the truth."

Where is the truth in food? Science. The truth is that all foods contain chemicals. Every piece you put in your mouth. Same with hormones, unless you're holding a salt shaker. These points are scientifically irrefutable. The facts are that we are all comprised of chemicals, and hormones are simply the chemical messengers of life. They aren't the bad guys, but the bullies certainly have done a successful job of crying wolf so much that the masses have come running.

"Free" doesn't mean natural. "Free" doesn't mean healthy. "Free" is not better. "Free" is marketing. It is difference without distinction. And why are you letting the bullies make you feel guilty with one word, anyhow?

Gluten-free

The "gluten-free" label is a slightly different case. It can be very helpful to the 0.5% of the population with celiac disease, who need to avoid gluten, a protein found in cereal grains, most commonly in wheat. Yet, 36% of food buyers search the label for gluten free information.[14] Gluten is the glue that makes dough elastic. Contrary to some claims, today's wheat doesn't contain more gluten, and there is no GMO wheat available on the market.[15]

Bullies play on your guilt over eating gluten and slap "gluten-free" labels on meat, water, almonds, and vegetables. It's akin to crying "wolf" for no reason, aside from sustaining a $6 billion gluten-free market with 20% of the population buying these products. If you're interested in learning more about gluten sensitivity and the value of grains, check out Chapter 30 of *Food Truths from Farm to Table*.

Preservative-free

The "preservative-free" and "additive-free" claims create an unnecessary fear of the wolf in the can or bottle. These claims also fly in the face of food science because preservatives and additives clearly protect the safety and taste of food—not to mention ensuring the availability of nutritious foods year-round. Think about how your great grandmother canned to preserve the summer's harvest, such as pickling cucumbers in a vinegar solution or making fruit jams with sugar. It's gone on for centuries; our ancestors preserved meat and fish with salt and added herbs to improve the flavor of foods.

Have you ever dropped apple slices in lemon juice water to prevent them from browning? That's an additive acting as a preservative. Did you know that preservatives, additives and colors are regulated by the Food and Drug Administration (FDA) before they are allowed to be added to food? FDA maintains a list of over 3000 ingredients, many of which you use at home, such as sugar, spices baking soda, salt, yeast, and colors.

The FDA reports, "When evaluating the safety of a substance and whether it should be approved, FDA considers: 1) the composition and properties of the substance, 2) the amount that would typically be consumed, 3) immediate and long-term health effects, and 4) various safety factors. The evaluation determines an appropriate level of use that includes a built-in safety margin—a factor that allows for uncertainty about the levels of consumption that are expected to be harmless. In other words, the levels of use that gain approval are much lower than what would be expected to have any adverse effect."[16]

However, supplements, now a $40 million business that has grown nearly tenfold in sales over the last 25 years, aren't regulated by the same stringent FDA standards. Perhaps we should look for dangers in our own shopping bags before buying into the wolf-claims.

HFCS-free

Likewise with the "HFCS-free" claim. High Fructose Corn Syrup (HFCS) is a sweetener. It is nearly identical to table sugar, honey, agave syrup, cane sugar, or maple syrup—all of which contain about the same amount of calories. If you're like me and have a wicked sweet tooth, you're trying to reduce your sugar intake.

Here's what you need to know: sweeteners are added to make food taste better. If a product has a sweetener in it and is labeled as HFCS-free, rest assured some other sort of sweetener—and resulting calories—is most likely present. In other words, sugar is sugar, no matter what pretty label a bully slaps on a sweetener.

Remember "Nobody believes a liar, even when he is telling the truth."

Is genetic engineering the ugly duckling?

Distrust also comes from that which we don't understand or appears different from what we consider normal. The Ugly Duckling spins the tale of a bullied victim who eventually finds himself a beautiful swan. GMOs, with their very own butterfly "non-GMO label," are often maligned, much like the ugly duckling. The key question is whether there is a beautiful swan that will eventually emerge from the dramatic folklore surrounding GMOs.

My Canadian farming friend Dale Leftwich shared with me his personal experience about the medical value of GMOs. His views stem not from the value of the crops he grew in his fields north of the border; rather, they are far more personal. Dale has a daughter who was diagnosed with diabetes at age seven. "Life is better because of a stable source of insulin from GMO bacteria that produce more reliable insulin. There's an abundant source of reliable, cost effective insulin due to GMOs for my daughter and other diabetics, rather than relying on animals."

Just like insulin from GMO bacterium was created to solve a problem, genetic modification of plants is generally used to solve a problem such as the ability to resist bugs, viruses, worms or to create healthier foods. Why haven't GMOs found their place as the swan in food marketing? My research shows that people are pretty freaked out about changing genetics.

Can genetics help humans?

Here's what you need to know; no one is sticking a syringe into a plant, tomato, or fruit—or crossing them with frogs, as some claim. Instead, amazing revolutionary science that will someday help humans cure cancer and eliminate malnutrition is being conducted. The science in moving a gene from a bacterium or another plant to make better food is actually pretty cool and more precise than traditional breeding. I like to say that "genes are the coolest ingredient on your plate." And before these scientific discoveries can be implemented, they must undergo a decades-long approval process.

GMOs are designed to solve specific problems, such as providing a source of consistent, allergy-free insulin for diabetics or helping prevent blindness from malnutrition. Here's the deal; the only GMO/Bioengineered foods currently approved by the United States Department of Agriculture (USDA) are alfalfa, Arctic apple, canola, corn, cotton, eggplant, papaya, pineapple, Innate potato, salmon, soybean, summer squash, and sugar beet. That's all![17]

History and extensive research show genetic improvements such as hybridization, genetic modification, gene editing, transgenics, gene silencing, and newer breeding techniques have proven benefits. Among them:

- increased consumer convenience: seedless fruits and apples/potatoes that don't brown
- more affordable food: more production per acre or per animal decreases costs
- greater medical options: today's insulin and extensive cancer research is a direct result of transgenics
- fewer allergens: research on tweaking genes for the proteins that cause peanut allergies
- better nutrition with leaner, higher protein: lower fat meats, more digestible milk, lower saturated fat soybean oil
- solutions to malnutrition: Vitamin A in rice, research on other foods like sorghum
- improved opportunity for small-scale farmers: drought resistant, hardier crops and animals
- reduced carbon emissions: fewer machinery passes through the field, higher production
- decreased use of insecticides: corn, eggplants, and others resistant to bugs don't need to be sprayed
- improved animal welfare: selection for disposition, calving ease and cattle without horns
- greater preservation of biodiversity: less land required with higher production

How do these "ugly ducklings" create so many emotions? Again, bullies prey on fear. Fear is created by distrust. And distrust comes from what you don't know. The more removed you are from a place, product, or practice—the more likely you are to fall for fairytales

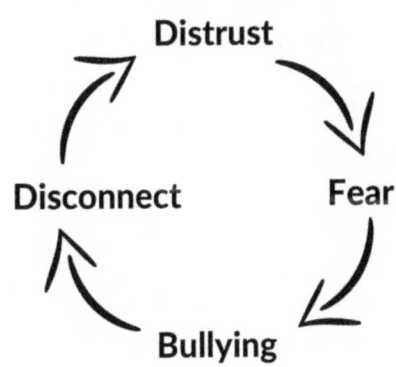

spun to help you feel good about your food. The GMO free or non-GMO label is especially dubious and confusing when used on products that have never had any genetically modified ingredients in them.

Canada implemented a national standard in to 2018 after complaints poured in about the non-GMO label: "If there aren't genetically-engineered varieties for a product's ingredient(s), you can't label it as non-GMO without a descriptor." For example, since there are no GMO peppers on the market, a non-GMO claim would have to state something along the lines of "like all peppers, these peppers are not a product of genetic engineering."[18]

You decide whether GMO fits your family's standards or not. Just know that the non-GMO butterfly flying through the grocery store may be the prettiest bully you come across, but it's not as beautiful as the swan of truth.

Difference without distinction

What's the best label for you to look for? B.S.-free! I'll provide you with more examples of B.S. and measurable labels in later sections. Avoid the fairytale of health halos, which are terms placed on food to lead you believe they are healthier. Free is not better. If there is no defined distinction that can be proven scientifically how one food is different than another, it's a fairytale.

Hormone hysteria is the next fairytale we'll look at on the playground of food bullying.

CHAPTER 6

Are hormones the wicked fairy or Sleeping Beauty?

Like many young girls, my daughter adored princesses and even wore sparkly dresses out to the barn. As a little girl, she was naturally drawn to the "tough" princesses like Pocahontas and Mulan, but she especially loved Sleeping Beauty in her sparkling yellow ball gown. I encouraged her to have brains, brawn, and grace; today she is an amazing student athlete who can wear two-inch heels and handle a ton of cow or a 5K race without blinking.

Because she used to love sleeping, I suspect her secret admiration for Sleeping Beauty was that century-long nap. Imagine that kind of sleep in your own life. Would it be caused by a food coma? Exhaustion? Hormones? Sleeping Beauty, which dates back to the 13th-century, was cursed by the wicked fairy who wasn't invited to Beauty's christening.

As the tale goes, everyone coddles young Beauty, sometimes known as Briar Rose. Then, on her 16th birthday, fate finds her, and off to sleep she goes.

Hormones are the chemical messengers required for life, found in every food, and should not be feared.

Ironically, Disney has created a few different movies featuring Sleepy Beauty but achieved much greater success with Maleficent, which retells Sleeping Beauty from the perspective of the vengeful fairy. Perhaps the negative, dark side is a whole lot more compelling?

Are hormones Maleficent or mainstream?

Similarly, consider the case of hormones in food; the "dark side" is a fairytale that is told with greater frequency. The Maleficent in this fairytale sounds like: "Food pumped full of hormones is causing cancer, early puberty, obesity, etc." As a mom, I understand why hormones freak parents out. They sound scary, but, in fact, hormones serve a natural purpose in all living things. They are the chemical messengers of life.

Given the hysteria around hormones in food, you may be surprised to learn about these comparisons of steroid levels in different foods, using standard serving sizes. Keep in mind that steroids are just the name of a class of hormones and these are not the muscle-pumping kind.

- Tofu naturally has 16,200,000 times more steroids than beef
- Pinto beans have 55,500 times more steroids than a glass of milk
- Peanuts have 28,000 times more steroids than eggs[19]

What about your hormones?

Love them or hate them, we can't exist without hormones; they are the chemical messengers of life. Consider birth control pills, testosterone therapy, and hormone replacement therapy. What hormone dosage are humans ingesting and how long does it stay in their system? As an example, let's say a 170-pound woman on low dose birth control takes about 0.48 milligrams (mg.) of estrogen monthly (not to mention the progesterone) for 21 of 28 days every month. If she—or anyone else on hormone therapy—stops taking it, does the hormone stop working?

Yes, hormones stop working if you no longer take them. Consider the consequences if a woman misses one day of birth control pills. Hormones don't pile up in your system; they do not have a build-up effect that prevents pregnancy, causes cancer, or turns you into the Incredible Hulk. The same is true in both humans and cattle. Hormones don't build up.

The truth about hormones in farm animals

It is true that some beef comes from cattle with hormone implants. It's similar to hormone replacement therapy used in humans, as it allows the animals to grow faster. The faster the animal grows, the less environmental impact. Using hormone implants is an environmentally important practice that reduces greenhouse gas emissions by approximately five percent.[20]

Why are cattle implanted with estrogen, testosterone, and progesterone? Because male calves are castrated to become steers and prevent aggression, they lose their hormone producing organ. Providing small amounts of these or similar hormones allows them to regain some of the growth rate they would naturally have as bulls. Further, implants, like human hormones, are actually naturally produced hormones.

The amounts of hormones in an implant are a fraction of the natural production of mature bulls or heifers. A 1,300-pound steer is implanted with 30 mg. of estrogen to last 150 days. And that's all the hormones he gets. Compare that to the estrogen in a typical birth control pill.

Implants have been used in beef cattle since 1954 because they also help reduce the carbon footprint of meat. Cattle with implants can convert their feed to muscle more efficiently and grow 15% faster during the finishing phase, which is when cattle are being prepared to provide the highest quality meat. More feed efficiency and faster growth mean less environmental impact.

How are these implants actually put in cattle? Implants are about the size of an Advil tablet and placed under the skin on the backside of the ear. The implant is put there because the ear never enters the meat supply. The animal never has hormones injected and extensive research shows hormone implants have no effect on beef quality, nutritional value, or safety.[19]

Some farmers and ranchers use implants and some do not, but now you can understand a bit more about the claim. The hormonal difference between beef produced with implants compared to non-implanted beef is two one-billionths of a gram, or two nanograms.[19]

What about chickens and pigs? As I wrote earlier, supplemental hormones are banned from use in poultry—whether in meat or eggs. The same is true of pigs, which means you've been wasting your money if you've been spending more for "no added hormones" labels on bacon, pork chops, eggs, turkey, chicken breasts, etc.

Is milk a hormone cocktail?

The dairy case is a fascinating case study in how people are being bullied into changing their food purchases. The hysteria around "hormones in dairy products" is a prime example. Labels are often used to convey a claim to alter the perception of the product, in order for the manufacturer and retailer to sell more and/or sell at a higher price.

Look no further than the fear mongering surrounding the protein hormone rBST, recombinant Bovine Somatotropin, which was approved by FDA in 1993 and entered the marketplace. I have personal familiarity with rBST from my days working as an undergraduate in the Animal Reproductive Physiology Laboratory. I assisted with some of the final experiments conducted at my alma mater, Michigan State University. In other words, I gave a whole lot of cows shots of rBST. I can confidently tell you from both personal experience and exhaustive research results that rBST does not harm cows and does not in any way adversely affect the quality of the milk they produce.

Why? Because BST naturally occurs in a cow's body. It's necessary for the production of milk—just like somatotropins are present in all animals (including women) with lactating capabilities. Somatotropin is a protein hormone that is important to support tissue health, growth and maintenance. Giving a cow a "booster" means she will make about 7% more milk—and will require more food to sustain the right body weight. The resulting milk is the same; there is no test that has identified additional hormone levels from cows given rBST. However, because of the backlash from rBST bullying, very few dairy farmers are allowed to use rBST today despite the management advantages the hormone provides.

Whether it's rBST or other hormones, it's important to understand that these hormones can be quite different from animals to humans. For example, our bodies don't even recognize rBST. The UN's Food and Agriculture Organization (FAO) has confirmed that the human and bovine receptors and hormones are different from one another.

You may also hear about insulin-like growth factor I (IGF-I), a protein hormone controlled by bST, being higher in cows given rBST. In fact, IGF-I levels in milk from rbST-supplemented cows fall within the normal range and are lower than levels found naturally in human blood and other tissues. It's important to understand this protein hormone is safe, even in high doses. Like any other dietary proteins, enzymes in your digestive tract break down all protein hormones—such as rBST and IGF-I—before you absorb it.

Now you know some of science related to the misleading "This milk was produced without rBST" claim on the milk jug label. Even the label that tells us that "There is no significant difference between milk derived from rBST-treated cows and non-rBST-treated cows" is unnecessary. And, on top of all of this, rBST is rarely used in the U.S. and not at all in Canada. The controversy that has been created is all about food bullying, driven by sales motives.

Does milk have hormones in it? Sure. Hormones like IGF-I support bone growth and are not found in "milk" derived from almonds or soybeans. Half of all men and 75% of women do not get adequate calcium in their diets. Both boys and girls do not get enough calcium, starting at age 19 and nine, respectively. Dairy products cannot be matched for the available calcium by other foods or supplements, regardless of label claims.

Do animal hormones cause early puberty?

I've never met a parent who doesn't worry about his or her children…especially when it comes to hormones. After all, who wants to deal with the frenzied chaos and emotions of puberty? The Academy of Nutrition and Dietetics (AND) reported that girls enter puberty today at a younger age than they did 30 years ago. There is debate as to how much earlier, but studies indicate it is about six months earlier.[21]

Some scientists believe the increase in childhood obesity may lead to earlier puberty. Dr. Frank Biro from the University of Cincinnati points out a fattier diet and more food may be largely responsible for girls developing earlier. Observational studies link higher body mass index or increased body fatness with earlier puberty. Puberty is the preparation of the body to begin supporting reproduction. A body that has received more nutrition over time reaches that point earlier. Fattier foods mean a body reaches that point earlier.

"Yes, children are exhibiting signs of puberty at an earlier age. There are several studies that have found that pubertal development has changed, but looking at the data, you can clearly see that this trend began decades before the use of hormones was introduced into agriculture, and is seen in countries where rbST was never introduced. So, hormones in meat or milk aren't to blame," according to Layla Katiraee of SciMoms blog.[22]

Bullies make hormones a best-seller

Looks like hormones are basically mainstream and not an evil Maleficent, even if they make for a best-selling, sensationalized fairytale. Stand up to the food bullies on this one; animals are not being pumped full of hormones to damage you or your family. Remember that nutrition, exercise, and fat and sugar intake likely have a lot more to do with early development in kids than hormones in food. And embrace hormones for the critical role they play in life!

Sustainability and the folklore around big versus small are up next.

CHAPTER 7

Is Jack or the giant a more sustainable farmer?

We love to cheer on the little guy, from David versus Goliath to Jack and the Beanstalk. The small, unknown school knocks out the well-known basketball powerhouse from the big NCAA tournament dance. A team from a tiny tropical country makes its first appearance in the Winter Olympics. After all, the little guy has an intrinsic disadvantage to overcome, right?

Not always, particularly when it comes to folklore around how food is raised. This is especially true when it comes to the debate related to farm size. A frequent, prevailing myth is that small farms are better than larger ones. We will take a look at that fairytales about farm size in this chapter, including the transitions family farms have had to make through the generations.

Just like Jack traded the family's only cow for handful of magic beans in Jack and the Beanstalk, farmers have had to adapt. Sometimes they switch to a specialization like omega-rich soybeans, white corn for tortillas, or hops for beer. Other farmers *There is no single "right" way to sustainably grow food.*

choose to increase their farm size so they have enough income to support their family and bring additional family members into the business. Yet others look to a niche market, such as Community Supported Agriculture (CSA). The outcome of these adaptions has been impressive; today's farmers and ranchers produce 262% more food with 2% fewer inputs compared to 1950, according to the American Farm Bureau Federation.

Keep in mind that most farmers are price takers, not price makers. In nearly every segment, they are told what their price will be—regardless of weather, cost of input products, and regulatory requirements. Farmers need to make enough income to support their family or it is not a sustainable business. In 2017, the USDA counted 12,000 fewer farms compared to the previous year and a million fewer acres of farmland. They estimated the total number of U.S. farms at 2.05 million and the total number of farm acres at 910 million. The average farm size is two acres bigger than a year prior, at 444 acres.

Is one size of farm right and the other wrong? Not necessarily, but food bullies frequently will spin folklore around larger "giant" farmers with labels such as "industrial agriculture" and "factory farming." It seems the inherent viewpoint is that small is better and big is bad, which is folklore. There is no single right way to grow food.

Are animals abused on large farms?

My family lives on a small farm; we personally care for our dairy animals, each of which has a name and is, frankly, spoiled rotten. We love them, but we also know their purpose is to provide humans with milk and meat. We consider it an honor and privilege to care for them so that they can provide us with food. That perspective is an important difference between farm animal owners and pet owners. In other words, my cow is not your dog.

Another David versus Goliath fairytale is that large farms abuse animals. After I've walked ranches covering tens of thousands of acres, been in pens that held thousands of animals, and watched hundreds of large animal farmers go about their work, this need to demonize larger farms and ranches mystifies me. The fact is, there is no one 'right way' to farm—and, yes, a few bad actors can be found on both the smallest and largest operations.

Research backs up my personal experience. "The size of a livestock feeding facility does not affect the quality of animal welfare." That according to research published by a United Kingdom-based, non-profit that examined the welfare level on 60 conventional pig farms in Northern Germany with capacity ranging from 250 to 11,000 pigs. In the report published in the journal *Animal Welfare*, co-author Dr. Christian Lambertz of the Research Institute of Organic Agriculture states "The study did not show that farm size was a factor for the animals' welfare." The researchers reported that none of the farm sizes proved superior in terms of animal welfare when measured on four basic principles— good feeding, good housing, good health, and appropriate behavior.[23]

Is "big" bad and "small" bucolic?

How can small, quaint farms be the heroes, while large, modern farms are the villain? Consider the long-term sustainability of a family business. As Wisconsin corn and soybean farmer Kevin Hoyer said, "Sustainability is multipronged. It's about improving upon what you have by positively influencing environmental, economic, and society factors. Overall sustainability can be found within all sizes of farms."

Modern farms that focus on high yield, such as feedlots, can use land more efficiently. For example, research, backed by several studies with a lot of data, suggests that "impacts on wild populations would be greatly reduced through boosting yields on existing farmland as to spare remaining natural habitats."[24] The article goes on to report that the overall negative environmental impact of lower-yield systems (those on smaller acreage or less efficient practices, such as organic) are underestimated. Unfortunately, the vast majority of media and environmental group attention has been focused on greenhouse gas emissions and nutrient losses on large farms.[24]

This notion that small farm operations are superior to large ones is also disproved if you look at the farms growing your fruits and vegetables. For them, the 2011 Food Safety Modernization Act (FSMA) increased the cost of food safety on the farm level due to requirements in paperwork, equipment, labor. These costs are often not reimbursed to farmers. When it comes to bearing the cost of following rules to keep your produce safe, the bigger the farm, the better, according to a 2018 USDA study. The very largest farms will spend 0.3% of their sales on food safety compliance, compared with 6.8% of sales for small farms.[25] In other words, the relative cost to small farms is twenty times greater than to large farms. That's an especially tough disparity with respect to profitability and sustainability of the family business.

Why the continued downward slide in the number of farms? There are many factors—from lower prices at the farm gate, an aging farm population, increased regulatory concerns, and environmental pressures. However, if a family is going to stay in the business today, they typically either become specialized or grow the size of their operation. Specialization frequently requires more labor, paperwork, and requirements from product buyers. Expansion often comes with more regulations, paperwork, and scrutiny. Both choices come with advantages and disadvantages.

There is no perfect farm size

Don't fall for the fairytales about farm size. There is no perfect size; all sizes and shapes of farms are needed to meet our nutritional needs. The same is true with food; there is no perfect food choice. Remember, the more removed you are from a place, product, or practice—the more likely you are to fall for fairytales spun to help you feel good about your food.

The next fairytale we'll explore is about the environmental folklore of meat and milk production.

CHAPTER 8

Are cow farts folklore?

If you've read my other books, you may remember Perfect, a cow who gave me many life lessons—and her descendants that grace our pasture today. Perfect had many ways to express her opinions, like farting after a good meal and belching loudly when she was happy. As anyone who has worked cattle can attest to, both cow farts and belches stink. Perfect's belching was passed on to great-great-great granddaughter Peppermint, who actually not only belched, but coughed up her entire cud on my daughter while they were working together preparing for a show. I found the whole smelly episode very amusing. Then Peppermint's daughter, Patience, did the same thing to me last summer. It was just gross, but my husband laughed as my hair blew back and regurgitated feed splatted on my face.

Cows = Recycling

You see, cattle are amazing recyclers, even if they do burp and fart. They're ruminants, meaning they have four special compartments in their stomach that allow them to digest food we cannot, recycling forages from

Eating meat and drinking milk are not environmentally irresponsible.

land that can't grow your food. What's really cool about ruminants is that they make use of land that would not be productive otherwise. As much as 70% of all agricultural land globally is range land that can only be utilized as grazing land for ruminant livestock, according to the Foreign Agricultural Organization (FAO) in 2013.

Why? Cattles' unique digestive system allows them to process grasses, hay, and corn—all of which are an important part of their diet. A key part of digestion is belching up their partially digested cud and chewing it. Perhaps gross, but it allows grass and protein to be converted into meat and milk. Amazingly enough, the FAO study also shows direct greenhouse gas emissions from U.S. livestock have declined 11.3% since 1961, while production of livestock meat more than doubled due to more efficient farming practices.

Please enjoy your meat without feeling like you are damaging the planet. Meatless Monday is a bit of a fairytale in itself because you're not going to save the environment by eliminating a key protein source one day of the week.

Animal agriculture decreases carbon footprint

Even if Americans eliminated all animal protein, it would only reduce greenhouse gas emissions by 2.6% in the U.S. There is actually a decreasing carbon footprint for animal agriculture, and this is a trend that will continue as long as livestock producers are allowed to improve their efficiency through modern technology.

"As the scale and impacts of climate change become increasingly alarming, meat is a popular target for action. Advocates urge the public to eat less meat to save the environment. Some activists have called for taxing meat to reduce consumption of it."[26]

Reality is that even if ALL Americans adopted Meatless Monday, there would only be a 0.5% impact. Personally, I choose protein and balanced nutrition over this nominal number. Make your choice according to your own standards, but know consumption of meat does not have massive environmental consequences.

What about your personal gases?

Generation of the electricity that powers houses like yours creates seven times more greenhouse gas emissions than the methane of ALL the livestock in the U.S., according to EPA, 2016. Humans need to take responsibility for the gases created by their lives before pointing the finger at meat and milk. All of agriculture accounted for 9% of U.S. greenhouse gas emissions (animal ag is only 3.9% of that), as compared to electricity production (28%) and industry (9%).[27]

Transportation in the U.S. also generates seven times more greenhouse gas emissions than methane from livestock—a fact that has always made me wonder why SUV-driving consumers, or even those in Camrys, raise questions about meat when drivers could lessen their personal impact far more quickly through a change in vehicles.

That's very different than the incorrect 2006 FAO report, "Livestock's Long Shadow," which armed environmental bullies and received widespread international attention. The grossly exaggerated figures around animal agriculture's impact were later corrected by the report's senior author Henning Seinfeld, but the damage from misinformation was already done.[28]

Sustainability is more than just the environment

Work has been ongoing to improve sustainability across the meat case, from beef to pork to turkeys. Wanda, a pork farmer from Minnesota, talked about the focus she and her family put on sustainability. "The technology is there to help us be more sustainable. Our hogs use less water and less food. Manure is recycled from under the barn, and it's a far better nutrient. It's the ultimate recycling program."

Another example is a Michigan turkey farm that powers 400 average American houses through used turkey litter that is burned to create electricity. The litter is the result of a clean waste system that results in a zero-carbon footprint. It's not folklore; many farms are amazing examples of creativity in solving problems that impact us all. Efforts will continue to be made to reduce agriculture's impact on the environment; be sure you're getting information from a farmer about this, rather than a bully.

Sustainability has both environmental and economic dimensions. It is not an either/or proposition. Sustainable practices encompass both dimensions, as well as a social dimension. Giving up meat will not save the climate, but eating meat does help family businesses and provides nutrition for your own family.

Personally, I believe it's wise to pick up a pork loin and some hamburger, turkey legs, lamb roast, or chicken breasts on every trip to the store because the nutrition provided by meat easily outweighs any negative environmental impact. My family needs that nutrition. And I won't let folklore sway my standards. How about you?

SECTION 3

Building your own story to understand food bullying

CHAPTER 9

Who are the players?

"That's smelly and disgusting." I have a confession; I am a food bully. So is my friend Hannah. Our husbands like to bait us with remarks about cooking corned beef hash. Hannah and I both hold a rather strong opinion that corned beef makes the kitchen smell horrible, and we spare no words in expressing our deep dislike of it. "Do not cook that in my kitchen," is our mantra.

Are you also a bully? Likely, we all are at some level.

Most of us don't intend to bully or be bullied. It's important we understand the elements of bullying, in order to overcome it and build our own food story. Section 3 will cover a lot about how our minds are manipulated around food. I've done my best to distill the psychology and science of what's happening to our brains in each of the six chapters, but be prepared for this section to be more complex. I know you can sort through it to better manage what's happening in your brain in order to make more rational decisions.

Eat your brussels sprouts!

A hog farmer in Ohio described his mom as a food bully. "She tried to make me eat

Who is influencing you through implied power of position, platform, or product?

those horrible brussels sprouts. I sat at the table for hours and never did eat them." We, as parents, are often bullies, even if it is with the best intentions.

An adoptive mom shared her story. "My daughter is now a more adventurous eater than me or her dad. But when she came to us, she was four months old and weighed 10 pounds. I started getting anxious and even angry at dinner, knowing it was going to be a fight to get her to eat.

"When I called the pediatrician, he gave me the best advice. He told me I was setting my daughter up for food problems and anxieties later in life, when her pickiness was really my problem— not hers. I was shocked, but began to realize I was making each dinner a time of anxiety for us both.

"I came away with an entirely new approach. I would always have two things she would eat, but I never made anything separate for her. Some nights she only ate rolls and fruit and nothing else, but as the doctor said, she would actually eat more if I changed my attitude. He was right. I was a food bully. I don't like to think of it that way, but I was." This baby boomer mom ended her story on a positive note, reporting that her now adult daughter happily eats a wide variety of cuisines.

In truth, parents have bullied for generations and likely will continue to do so. They are in the position of power and therefore have significant influence over food decisions. At least until the child falls in love with chocolate or Cheetos.

However, parents represent just one example among many as we consider who the players are on the food bullying playground. In the remainder of this chapter, we will consider several other players in the context of "implied power."

What is implied power?

A celebrity TV chef has implied power; he doesn't necessarily say this, but his position and celebrity status imply power that can extend to recommendations well beyond how to create a food dish. Again, the chef's power is implied by his or her position, platform, or product. It may be expressed verbally, in writing, artfully, or via body language. And it can start with the best of intentions, then turn toward bullying.

For example, a doctor can be a very positive influence toward healthy living, but she becomes a bully when suggesting people shouldn't eat GMOs because of farming practices. A conventional farmer is a positive influence in discussing her sustainability practices, but she becomes a bully when condemning a consumer or another farmer who chooses organic.

As adults, we have control over our food choices, but we are certainly influenced by people, causes, and products. It's important to note that no one has any real power over us. I like to say "the attention goes where your energy flows." If you closely follow a chef or doctor, you're likely to given more credence to their recommendation. The power implied by one's position, platform, or product can start with the best of intentions, then turn to bullying, even if it's not intentional.

In other words, bullying begins where firsthand expertise ends. Unfortunately, in today's overly sensationalized food playground, there are many who bully through their implied power—whether it is position, platform, or product. I've created the table below to outline the three categories of implied power and will provide examples in the subsequent sections.

Implied Power	Description	Examples on food playground
Position	*People whose career or expertise gives implied power over others' choices.*	*Teachers, doctors, nurses, politicians, chefs, fitness instructors, dietitians, farmers*
Platform	*People whose bully pulpit gives them implied power over others.*	*Friends, celebrities, colleagues, social media connections, journalists, gym nutritionists, activists, parents*
Product	*Items whose claims, market share, labels give them implied power.*	*Manufacturers, grocery stores, restaurants, brands marketers, pyramid marketing products, fitness products, supplements*

Do they really know food and farming?

Consider this scenario from an Indiana classroom. The 12-year-old, twin son and daughter of one of my closest friends had some serious questions about their food after watching a video in a seventh-grade social studies class at a middle school in an upper-class suburb. While corn and soybeans were being harvested around the school, the teacher featured a food marketing video during their social studies class. There was not a debate, or a discussion on critical thinking, only the sensationalized video.

These twins have followed my daughter around our pasture since they were all toddlers, they know our cattle by name, and they even helped bring one of our newborn calves home in the back of their van. But they now question what farmers are doing to animals after hearing "cows don't ever see grass, chickens are injected with hormones, and pigs are kept inside." How is this part of their education?

Why would a teacher put those ideas into their heads with blatant marketing propaganda from a restaurant with a questionable track record? There was no debate, no other side presented, no lesson in marketing. The result? Kids feeling bad about their food and questioning farming. It broke my heart to hear these questions from children whom I once held in my hand when they were born very prematurely and spent months in the NICU. When we sat down for dinner, I first asked them what video it was, and when I heard it was from Chipotle, I somehow managed to resist banging my head on the table in frustration over the obvious bullying through implied power.

"Why do you think a food company would make a video?" I asked them as gently as I could. They said, "to show bad things farmers do." I pressed a little further and asked what a restaurant wanted to do. "Sell food!" they agreed. "So do you think they might be telling lies to sell more food?" was my response, quickly followed by "have you ever seen us abuse our animals or do anything mean to them?" They shook their heads while joyfully telling stories of the animals they've watched us raise through the years. I then asked if they thought our cattle were the same as their dogs; we all agreed that farm animals have a different purpose than pets.

"It's illegal to give chickens hormones," I next explained, along with the fact that there are no such products available. They wanted to know why chickens were so big, wondering if I was sure chickens were not pumped full of something. So, we got into a discussion about genetics and the fact that chickens have been bred to have bigger breasts because that's what people like to eat.

Their parents chimed in as we discussed why pigs stay inside. We talked diseases, predators, and huge swings in temperature. I told them it was really sad that a marketing company was telling lies about farmers. The whole conversation gave me a sick feeling.

Ideas planted by teachers last a lifetime, whether good or bad. Marketing and bias don't belong in the classroom; science and well-rounded debate do. Teacher bias deserves even more attention than journalistic bias because young students can't simply 'turn off' their education the way so many adults have silenced the news.

We need to educate students in critical thinking skills, covered in Chapter 18—not fill them with dubious or patently false marketing messages. Shouldn't we be questioning teachers and professors who promote their own agenda in a classroom? I'm sure the teacher in question was an expert in social studies, but that expertise does not extend to firsthand experience in farming or nutrition choices. Regardless, he influences his classes through implied power of position. The same applies to college campuses and professors' influence over students.

Have you experienced this in your own education? What about with doctors, nurses, or fitness instructors? Are they making recommendations around food and food production without firsthand knowledge? Remember, bullying stemming from the power of position often begins where firsthand expertise ends.

Does the authority figure have any firsthand experience with how food is raised or formal education concerning farming? Likely not. However, she holds a position that gives implied power over others' food choices, including making recommendations about "right" farming practices and nutrition

What are they selling?

The "Dirty Dozen," a celebrity list of fruits and vegetables that you should <u>never</u> buy unless they're organic, is published by activists at the Environmental Working Group (EWG), who relies on the list for publicity to grow their platform. Turns out the real dirt is the activist group behind the Dirty Dozen list. Seventy nine percent of members of the Society of Toxicology rating EWG reports that the group overstates the health risk of chemicals.[29]

Many consumers believe the misinformation—and follow EWG's command that they must buy only organic versions of any foods on the Dirty Dozen list. This is a case study for the implied power of platform—an activist organization using social media to promote a controversial position and selling it as truth or even science. The result is, at a minimum, that many parents reading this misinformation feel guilty for not buying organic. Worse still, misinformation like this causes consumers to purchase and eat less produce at a time when 9 out of 10 people do not get enough fruits or vegetables. If you are concerned, please use the Safe Fruits & Veggies Calculator at http://safefruitsandveggies.com.

Can't we all agree that guilt should never replace nutrition on the plate? In a study of low-income shoppers, organic fruits and vegetables were preferred, but cost was a significant barrier against purchasing them. Even when this group was given science-based information about organic and conventional fruits and vegetables, they weren't more likely to buy more produce. Instead, misinformation, such as the Dirty Dozen list, identifying specific fruits and vegetables produced with pesticides made low income shoppers less likely to purchase any type of produce.[30]

Food choices are also influenced by the implied power of bloggers and others with a strong social media following, such as Food Babe. Her credentials? She started eating differently and lost weight, then blogged about it. Vani Hari, the Food Babe's real name, provides her website readers with no educational background or scientific credentials in dietetics, or food production and processing. She now uses her website for selling items such as meal plans, juicing blenders, and the "Food Babe Way," as well as specializing in creating fear about food through her "investigations."

While I agree we could all better understand what is in our food, I do not find it ethical to bully consumers and food companies, or to encourage an "army" to do so when there is no scientific evidence involved. In Hari's words, "Companies have no choice but to respond to us and improve the quality of their products." She proudly lists her fear mongering successes on her site, e.g., strong-arming Chick-Fil-A into announcing a plan to use antibiotic-free chickens in 2011, convincing Kraft to change its Mac and Cheese recipe, and inflaming people about Starbucks' Pumpkin Spice Latte.

Hari is clearly gifted at creating headlines, but an online blogger selling products does not have a better understanding of food ingredients than food scientists, microbiologists and the FDA. There's an extensive approval process and database of ingredients, which a person with firsthand expertise can explain. Instead, fear is created through a blogger's platform.

A fellow professional speaker from Canada points to her social media connections as people "armed with pseudo-science spreading lies aggressively about food production; they don't understand the consequence of their plans to eradicate GMOs or make the world organic, especially for hungry people."

In today's age of social media, activism has reached new heights. My company's research shows activists such as Greenpeace and the Humane Society of the United States (HSUS) growing their social media community more than 500-fold in the last 10 years.

Unfortunately, there are many who work to influence others through their implied power of platform on today's noisy food playground. Your friends may be as guilty of bullying through their Facebook posts proclaiming the value of drinking vinegar or sharing an article condemning the treatment farm animals, but do they have firsthand farming or nutrition expertise?

Is one food superior and the other inferior?

Chipotle's former "Food with Integrity" slogan is an example of this implied power of product, using misleading claims inferring their product is superior. Chipotle's website boasted that "since we opened the first Chipotle restaurant more than 22 years ago, we have served fresh, wholesome ingredients prepared using classic cooking techniques. It's always been a top priority to make sure that our delicious food is safe to eat."

Really? Let's take a look at the burrito chain's history of foodborne illness, including the recent outbreaks of clostridium in 2018 and norovirus in 2017. And these came after a rather infamous 2015 of foodborne illnesses that left five people sick from E. coli in Seattle, 234 sick in California from Norovirus, and 64 people sick from Salmonella in Minnesota. Then in the last quarter of 2015, 60 people got sick from E. coli in twelve states across the U.S. after eating at Chipotle. The last one in December 2015 sickened 151 people in Boston and led to the closing of that location.[31]

Do hundreds of people getting sick really square with Chipotle's "Food with Integrity" promise that was made in the same timeframe? The evidence clearly suggests not. And, besides, does your food truly have more integrity than mine? Sounds like bullying, as they often infer that modern-day farms are inferior, but then make people sick despite their "Food with Integrity" marketing mantra. It's an example of a food company's branding campaign leading you to believe its product is superior to increase its profits through increased sales. This is bullying using the implied power of product.

In short, a restaurant selling food should not be able to leverage implied power via misleading claims about their brand or product. Stand up to this sort of bullying; remember that food safety has to trump marketing at every meal in every restaurant or deli.

The same is true in the grocery stores, where some brands imply superiority. Whole Foods, an Austin-based company now owned by Amazon, is unquestionably big business with 89,000 employees in 490 stores in the U.S., Canada, and the United Kingdom. Whole Foods realized a cool $2.88 billion in profits in

2017.[32] Their sales flyers feature more food marketing claims than actual names of food, such as "Responsibly Farmed" and "Animal Welfare Rated," are just two examples of B.S. labels.

If your standards align with Whole Foods, what they like to call "America's Healthiest Grocery Store," and you can afford to shop there, please do so. Just know those standards aren't all about wholesome food, but include financial incentives. It's hypocritical to suggest otherwise. I also question what makes one grocery store brand healthier than another.

It's also unfair to imply food from this brand or any other is superior and to look down your nose at another parent who doesn't bring a Whole Foods bag for classroom snacks. After all, perhaps she doesn't buy into the implied power of product—or she just can't afford to do so.

Naming the bullies

This chapter has focused on the various players on the food bullying playground. These players constitute the "Who" dimension of the bullying story. Understanding who the players are is the first step in understanding all the aspects of bullying. There are hundreds of names, organizations, brands, individuals, and companies that could be listed. It's important to remember that the truth is often found in the middle, not in polarizing viewpoints.

Step back and ask yourself how these players can leverage implied power to bully you. Is the influence coming from position, platform, or product? Some bullies have figured out how to leverage all kinds of implied power, using position, platform, and product. As soon as you can identify who might bully you, regardless of intentions, you can begin building your plan to overcome food bullying.

Next we will take a look at identifying and understanding the motivators behind bullying.

CHAPTER 10

What are the motivators?

Jennifer Garner's favorite pet chicken tried to kill her new chicks. The actress keeps hens at her home, and, when she added to their flock last year, there were some problems. After all, chickens will be chickens; Captain Hook apparently didn't like her territory invaded and turned on the newcomers.

Garner told talk show host Ellen DeGeneres: "They're such nice pets until they get mad at each other. We had six chickens, we got seven new ones…we tried to introduce them, and Captain Hook, one of our older chickens, was not nice. She started trying to attack and kill the new chickens, specifically Henniker, so we got a small coop to protect the new ones." Garner even admitted to having a pep talk with Captain Hook, but it hasn't changed the hen's ways; she still wants to attack.

This should not come as a surprise. Farm animals follow a pecking order, even if they hang out in the backyard of a celebrity's home. Chickens are carnivores and cannibals, not to mention scavengers. They will do whatever it takes to survive.

Influence can change to bullying when food claims target your need for belonging and esteem.

Hardwired for survival

Like chickens, humans are hardwired for survival. Yet most messaging we receive around food has little to do with surviving—or even safety—but it is important to remember that nourishment is one of our most basic needs. It is the most basic of all of the needs this chapter addresses.

A formerly homeless woman in Massachusetts recently gave me a poignant reminder about how a person's very survival can be threatened on the playground of food bullying. "Real people are being harmed as the cost of food is manipulated by special interest groups. Thank you for your work and please thank farmers for theirs (from a mom who knows what hunger looks and feels like)."

She gave birth to her son when she was homeless. Can you imagine trying to feed a newborn in such an environment? Few of us understand real hunger, but, sadly enough, one in eight people in the U.S. and Canada live without food security. It's a reminder that the argument around food most often comes from a privileged position of food availability. People who live in conditions of chronic hunger and malnutrition worry more about their next meal than the latest label claim or what brand of food their friends recommend. Let's all remember that.

Is your trust misplaced or abused?

Sometimes our trust is misinformed, such as when Jennifer Garner trusted that Captain Hook would warmly welcome Hennifer to Garner's backyard chicken flock. Other times, trust is abused by the players on the food bullying playground, similar to Captain Hook abusing the new chickens in her role as the "queen" hen. As described in the last chapter, we typically trust those with implied power of position, platform, or product.

Before we examine needs, let's remember that we all purchase food, and we make those buying decisions on information we trust. It can be hard. For example, trust in a label that claims "all-natural" is misplaced because there is no standardization or scientific oversight to prove this claim. It is B.S. "All-natural" corn chips are likely equally as healthy as "all-natural" hot dogs. But if your Facebook friend convinces you that all-natural corn chips are a diet must-have and that kiddos at your backyard barbecue deserve all-natural hot dogs, are you bullied through implied power of platform? Again, trust can be misplaced, even in those we love.

Your trust is abused when a manufacturer attempts to label a product to stand out from similar products, all in the pursuit of money and/or power. A food company's marketing team decides labeling their meat "antibiotic-free" will differentiate their product in the very competitive meat case, resulting in more sales for the "antibiotic free" meat. The label infers superiority when, in fact, each brand of meat is tested equally for antibiotic residues. On a quick trip to the grocery store, it is easy to be bullied by the implied power of product and have your trust abused by label claims.

Chain of command

Let's take a look at the chain of command for our basic human needs, so we can determine where trust in food claims can be placed. These needs provide motivation for doing something, especially those reasons that are hidden or not obvious. Maslow's "Hierarchy of Needs" is arguably the best-known and most widely accepted theory of human motivation. Maslow's hierarchy demonstrates there are five, interdependent levels of basic human needs (motivators) that must be satisfied in sequence.

The hierarchy shows physiological needs must be met first, followed by our safety needs, then come belonging and esteem needs, and finally our need for self-actualization, which is key in reaching our highest potential. According to Maslow, all human actions can be largely explained based on these five levels of needs.

In my own research and work experience, I have increasingly found what I believe are close parallels between Maslow's hierarchy and what motivates both food sellers and food buyers (see chart below). By better understanding the motivation behind selling and buying behavior, we can also better grasp food bullying strategies, recognize when they are being used, and develop our own plans for resisting the mind games.

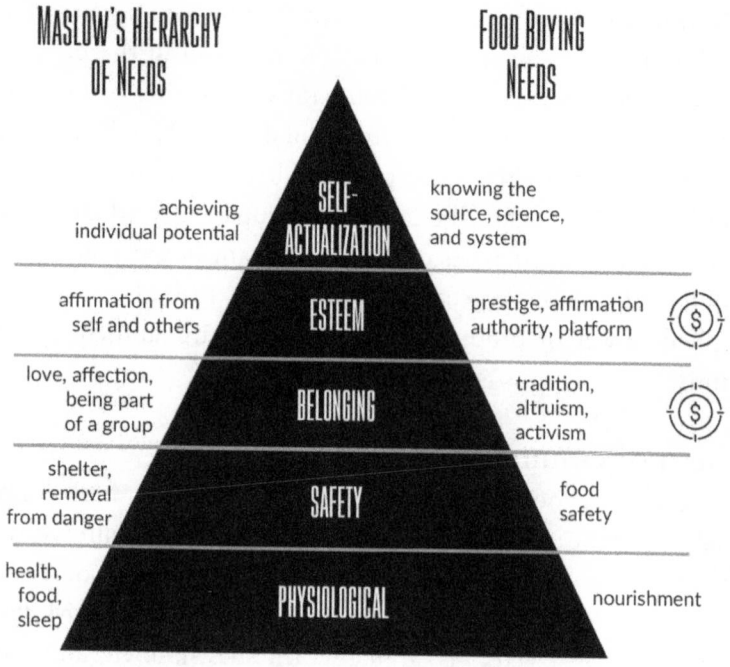

MASLOW'S HIERARCHY OF NEEDS

FOOD BUYING NEEDS

Maslow's Hierarchy of Needs	Level	Food Buying Needs
achieving individual potential	SELF-ACTUALIZATION	knowing the source, science, and system
affirmation from self and others	ESTEEM	prestige, affirmation authority, platform
love, affection, being part of a group	BELONGING	tradition, altruism, activism
shelter, removal from danger	SAFETY	food safety
health, food, sleep	PHYSIOLOGICAL	nourishment

Bullying most often preys on esteem and belonging needs, once the physiological and safety needs are met. I have also found that those selling food move from influence to bullying by focusing on our belonging and esteem motivations. By placing food buying needs on Maslow's hierarchy, we have a tool to understand and evaluate how motivation is used and abused across the food playground.

Influence changes to bullying

Looking at food buying needs on Maslow's hierarchy allows us to start with the fundamentals. The influence at the physiological and safety level is: "What is nutritious and safe?" Unfortunately, these two basic levels are often overlooked in developed countries; nutritious and safe food is largely assumed, even expected.

Moving up the hierarchy, influence can change to bullying in order to meet a buyer's belonging and esteem needs, as shown in these examples.

- Concern around food often starts from the interest in helping people—altruism, but a person who believes her way is the only way can turn into a zealot (the first level of food bullying).
- A farmer insistent on preserving a farming tradition that has been maintained for four generations can cause that farmer to judge other farmers who choose to change practices.
- An animal lover motivated by belonging may turn to activism and, consequently, shaming others who make different eating choices.
- A final example of influence turning to bullying: companies targeting the prestige need may try to build their customers' esteem by evangelizing to push groupthink.

The big business of food

As demonstrated on *Food Bullying's* model of food buying needs, the middle two levels are most frequently targeted for bullying, very often driven by those seeking profit. Food is big business; grocery stores, restaurants, drug stores, convenience stores, and mass merchandisers sold $5.75 trillion worth of food in 2017. That's more than twice the size of India's economy.[33]

Most Americans seemingly like visiting the grocery, averaging about 1.6 trips per week in 2018. Even though online grocery shopping has existed for years, the vast majority of consumers still prefer to buy groceries in stores. Walmart alone sold more than $318 billion in 2018, operating 4,761 stores nationwide, excluding Sam's Club.[34] There are now over 30,000 dollar stores, more than the six largest U.S. retailers combined (Walmart, Kroger, Costco, Home Depot, CVS, and Walgreens).[35] That's a lot of opportunity for Bull Speak!

Competition for food is intense, as is the need to differentiate products and/or brands. One manufacturer, talking off-the-record, noted "we could spend $100 million to educate people to accept our product or give them what they want on the label and we make $20 million."

As this example shows, it is common for food bullies to prey on people's fears to make money. Just over 5% of disposable income is spent on food at home and 4.7% is spent on food away from home, according to the USDA. If 10% of your income is being spent on food, isn't it important for you to be able to identify what motivators are targeted to get your money?

The many ways marketers appeal to your needs are overwhelming and complicated because they bring their own needs into it. Use this hierarchy of food buying needs to get back to the core question: "Is this food nutritious and safe?"

You will find it saves a lot of time, confusion, and guilt in the grocery store. Next, place food claims on the blank lines provided for the various levels of the hierarchy below to help identify potential bullying starting at the base of the food buying needs hierarchy. We'll work our way up the model with examples from each level and need. Feel free to fill in the blanks about where you think food claims fit.

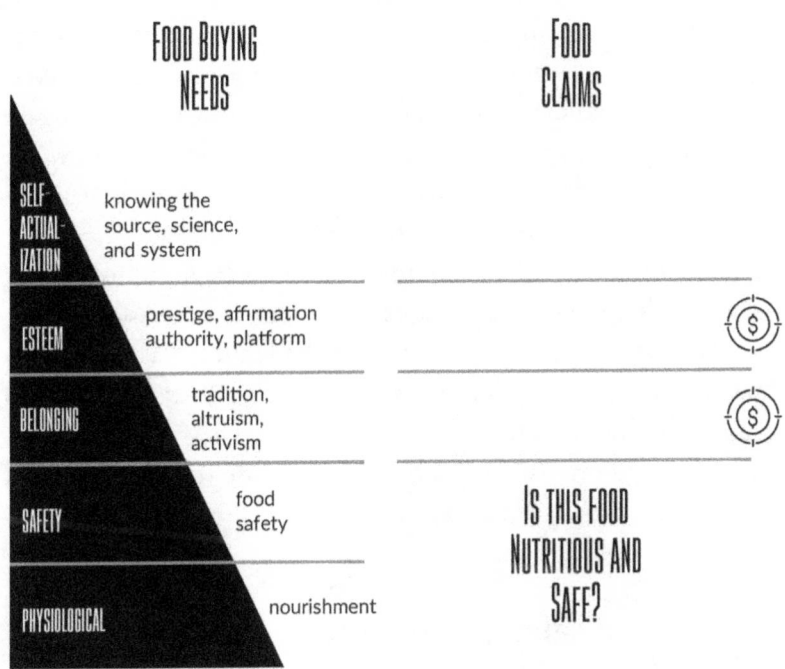

Physiological: Nourishment is a necessity

Is food available? Nourishment, or overcoming hunger, is one of our most basic needs. I've had the honor of working on food and agricultural issues around the world, which has provided a unique lens on meeting hunger needs. Visiting South Africa is a memory I'll carry for the rest of my life, especially the eyes of hungry children. Children who live in squatters' camps by the millions. Children who live in shacks that make an outhouse look like a condominium and play next to bootlegged raw electrical lines. Children who don't care about the politics of food, but only where they can find some nourishment.

I've seen those same desperate eyes in begging Egyptian children and in the Ukraine, shortly after communism fell. Then back in Indiana when my daughter started school and had hungry classmates who couldn't concentrate in class. The debate we have around food in developed countries is a very privileged one. It is one of my standards to always be mindful of those living in hunger, a perspective I wish more Americans held. Somehow, on the playground of food bullying, it is more righteous to debate the politics of food than the very real problem of hunger.

Even in the U.S., 12.5 million children were food insecure in 2017. That's enough hungry kids to fill city of Los Angeles! The Food and Agriculture Organization of the United Nations (FAO) reports 821 million undernourished people globally in 2017, up from 804 million in 2016.[36]

Before you evaluate any label claim, realize that the food you hold in your hand is a privilege many in the world do not have—including people in your hometown.

Safety: Food safety is invisible

Is the food safe? Once we meet our need for nourishment, food safety is the next need on the hierarchy. Our eating choices move up the food buying hierarchy if we're privileged enough, but safety comes first once the nourishment need is met. We are terrified of unsafe food, yet we live in a society where only 5% of people who use the bathroom wash their hands sufficiently enough to kill illness-causing germs.

Food marketers can take advantage of our intrinsic need for safety, like a 2018 Juice Press marketing campaign that featured hazmat-suited, gas-mask wearing people demonizing non-organic produce and creating fear in consumers. In an attempt to differentiate their product and tell customers that their juice was organic, they used scary images and language, such as "You'd be drinking genetically modified rank s#*t-tasting dead juice that smelled like fu#%ing poison."[37] Vulgar fear mongering like this is not only deception, it preys on your need for safety.

Food safety, at its best, is invisible. Consider reaching in the dairy case to grab a gallon of milk. While you will likely never think about it, the refrigeration of the case is checked regularly to ensure the safety of that milk, even though your gallon may sit for an hour in your hot car on the way home. And that milk goes through a whole lot of steps to be sure it's safe for you.

Did you know The FDA Grade A Pasteurized Milk Ordinance, started in 1924 and revised in 2009, has a legal standard requiring milk to contain no detectable antibiotics when tested with approved methods? If you're buying milk in the grocery store, the only kind you're purchasing is Grade A. While you will likely never see it, milk is tested multiple times to ensure no milk enters the food supply with antibiotics in it.

If a cow has to be treated with antibiotics to help her overcome infection, the milk is withheld from the human food supply for a FDA-mandated period of time. After that, the milk is tested to be sure it is clear before it goes from the cow through a milking machine to a bulk tank, where it is chilled. Milk samples are taken from each farm's bulk tank for antibiotic residue testing before being loaded on to a tanker. Every tanker of milk in the United States is also tested before the milk is pumped from the tanker for delivery at the processing plant. If the milk passes the test, it is pumped into the plant's holding tanks for processing, e.g., pasteurization, homogenization, or being turned into cheese, ice cream, yogurt, etc.

If milk does not pass antibiotic testing at the farm, the entire tanker load of milk is discarded. Farm samples are then reviewed to find the source of the antibiotic residues. The farm is usually held financially responsible for the cost of the tanker load. Fines can be levied, and the processor may refuse shipment in the future. The veterinarian for the farm is also contacted and may be put under review by the FDA. As any dairy farmer or veterinarian will tell you, antibiotics are NOT something they take lightly.

You likely will never see these invisible steps, but all are in place for real food safety.

You are more likely to hear about recalls, particularly produce recalls, than the amazing tools in place to test your food. The FDA reported 1,928 recalls in their 2018 fiscal year. The scale of the recalls made many people worry about the safety of their food; recalls of eggs, pre-cut melons, ground beef, breakfast cereal, and romaine lettuce understandably led to many consumer questions and concerns. However, keep in mind that our ability to detect them has greatly improved, especially in recent years.

It turns out that the genetic technology so many fear, whole genome sequencing, is helping us have safer food. The bacteria responsible for many outbreaks mutate very quickly, which makes for a 'genetic fingerprint' that's easy to trace. Experts are now using genome sequencing, which relies on the DNA fingerprint of the food, to help determine its source. Pulsenet, a national laboratory network at the Center for Disease Control, uses that DNA fingerprint to link illnesses to one another and try to determine the source of the contamination.[38]

In other words, the same genetic technology that led to GMOs has rapidly increased detection rates for the organism making us sick and has allowed food safety experts to identify problems much earlier. That leads to safer food for you and me, even though whole genome sequencing is invisible to us.

Rather than assuming food is produced unsafely or falling victim to marketing campaigns that make you fear the safety of your food, stay mindful of the largely invisible world that ensures your food safety.

Belonging: Altruism

What about the friend who bullies without knowing it? She wants to save everyone and truly believes her way of eating will protect the world from all illness. It puts her stress over-the-top as she worries about people she loves being sick "when all they would have to do is eat correctly." Can you think of a time when you had the best of intentions, but likely bullied someone else?

Altruism, the need to help others, often drives us to bullying because we care too much. The intention is to help a friend or family member, to cure what ails them. We want our loved ones to live long, healthy, happy lives. Many times, this prompts many food fears, and sometimes leads to obsession, food paranoia, and worshiping a particular eating choice. The bully doesn't know he or she is bullying, and the victim (usually a friend or family member) can feel inferior, insulted, and guilty.

How can you share expert food information to help a person who really wants to help others?

Belonging: Tradition

"Don't eat what your grandma would not recognize" and "Don't eat what you can't pronounce" are messages promoted by some food elitists. Would you eat or cook with a product that contained ingredients like "amino acids, phenylalanine, octadecenoic acid, sugars, colors E160c and E306, flavors phenyl acetaldehyde and acetone—also contains benzene and sulfur?" Rest assured, your grandma used this food—eggs. The same with blueberries, which have the following ingredients: "sugars made up of 48% fructose, fatty acids like linoleic acid, flavors ethyl ethanoate and hydroxyl linalool, and colors E163a and E163e".

Australian chemistry teacher James Kennedy wanted to dispel a myth that chemicals are bad for us, so he created these ingredient lists. Most would never recognize a particular food item by its list of ingredients and, if you're like me, you trip over your tongue even in trying to pronounce them. But keep this example in mind when you hear messages appealing to your tradition need.

The need for tradition runs deep in families. For example, we always bake homemade cinnamon rolls to give as gifts at

Christmas, just as I was raised. My husband's Norwegian family makes Krumkake. Many holiday and family traditions center around food. It's not likely those traditions are going to change, but there are bullying messages targeting our need to honor traditions.

Food marketing tends to play on the idea that it was so much better when our grandparents were cooking and farming, in spite of significant improvements in food safety, animal welfare, and sustainability. How are bullies leveraging your need for tradition?

Belonging: Activism

"The company wants antibiotic-free, and they're willing to pay for it. But that means when turkeys get sick, I have to watch a percentage of them die. Plus, sick turkeys use more feed and grow slower, which increases the carbon footprint." This is from a turkey farmer, in response to Subway's demands for antibiotic-free turkeys. All of this is due to activist pressure from the U.S. Public Interest Research Group, who led the campaign to bully Subway.

Activists target restaurants, manufacturers, and grocery chains to carry their message. By bullying through the need for belonging, activists force their viewpoint on brands, which has a ripple effect across the food system. Consider these examples and how caving to activist pressure increased the carbon footprint, food waste, food costs, and B.S.

Who wants to eat a bruised potato? Not many. Rejection of brown potatoes can create food waste, which is a shame when a staggering 40% of food in the U.S. is wasted. Yet, McDonald's rejected the new Innate variety of potato in 2014 due to pressure from the activist group Food and Water Watch. The potato is resistant to bruising and browning, which Food & Water Watch claims is a threat to public health, in spite of years of rigorous research and hefty government approval.

Wendy's and Gerber both made it clear they also had no interest in the first genetically modified apple released, after strong-arming from Friends of the Earth. This is another product resulting from the gene silencing technology—the same technology that is being used to explore cures to illnesses such as cancer.

Many food manufacturers have been forced to make claims about how farm animals should be housed, claims driven by the Humane Society of the United States (HSUS) agenda. While many believe the organization is about local animal shelters, HSUS does not own, operate, or lease a single animal shelter in this country. They have worked diligently to mandate requirements about how pigs and chickens must be housed, increasing our food costs while—ignoring those with firsthand expertise, farmers.

Many people become activists to make the world a better place. I'm all for that, but be aware of activism eroding truth about your food—and of creating negative consequences related to animal welfare, the environment, and food price. In my experience, truth comes from those with firsthand experience, not activists.

Esteem: Authority

Panera Bread, claims on its food menu that "100% of our food is 100% clean-eating." What exactly does that mean? Isn't clean a term that should be reserved for the laundry? Or the dishes? Or the windows? Does clean food mean that it's been washed? Or that the Panera employees washed their hands? Or is it implied superiority about the food itself?

What is Panera Bread's motivation? After sales of $7.5 billion in 2017, the restaurant chain is clearly focused on profitability across its 2,000 locations.[39] Panera, instead of using FDA or USDA standards, devised its own system to define standards of "clean." Is Panera's motivation authority or prestige through pushing their "clean" agenda? Are they appealing to people's esteem or trying to position Panera Bread as authority? Or maybe both? You decide, but please know terms such as "clean food" are bullying. I used to love Panera Bread, but I can no longer stomach their evangelizing and won't eat there anymore.

Some people and brands want to be considered an authority, which I believe has led to more confusion. When you consider authority claims, be sure to look for measurable and meaningful labels, not marketing claims.

Esteem: Affirmation

"I think people are very fearful and being rigid around food choices is one way to control anxiety and reassure themselves that they are doing the right thing," noted Leia Flure, a dietitian in Illinois. How do labels on food packages and restaurant menus appeal to our need for affirmation?

The need for esteem looks different to parents who don't have enough to make ends meet. According to a sociology researcher at Stanford, "For parents raising their kids in poverty, having to say "no" was a part of daily life. Their financial circumstances forced them to deny their children's requests—for a new pair of Nikes, say, or a trip to Disneyland—all the time. This wasn't tough for the kids alone; it also left the poor parents feeling guilty and inadequate.

"Compared to all the things poor parents truly couldn't afford, junk food was something they could often say 'yes' to. Poor parents told me they could almost always scrounge up a dollar to buy their kids a can of soda or a bag of chips. So, when poor parents could afford to oblige such requests, they did.

"Honoring requests for junk food allowed poor parents to show their children that they loved them, heard them, and could meet their needs. As one low-income, single mother told me: 'They want it, they'll get it. One day they'll know. They'll know I love them, and that's all that matters.'

"Junk food purchases not only brought smiles to kids' faces, but also gave parents something equally vital: a sense of worth and competence as parents in an environment where those feelings were constantly jeopardized."[40]

Food can be affirmation, both positive and negative. Health halos are another form of affirmation; some people think they're doing you a favor by telling you that your food is killing you. In reality, they're affirming their value and worth. Remember, you can agree to disagree.

Rather than looking to food for affirmation, remember to get back to the basics: "Is it safe and nutritious?"

Esteem: Platform

Consider Gwyneth Paltrow's rather eccentric recommendations, such as telling women to steam their vagina or drink goat's milk for a week straight to remove parasites. You may consider it gross (as do I), but she says, "I can monetize those eyeballs," referring to her interest in growing a bigger platform for greater influence and sales.[41] Like food safety, monetization of misinformation is invisible. Many celebrities make sensationalized claims or appeal to your need for esteem because they want to grow their platform and line their pockets.

The same is true for a medical doctor who has been called before Congress. The Doctor Oz Show is one of the top U.S. talk shows, hosted by Dr. Mehmet Oz. "Cancer," he told the New Yorker, "is our Angelina Jolie. We could sell that show every day." As a person who has taken care of a loved one with cancer, I don't know which is sadder—that people are "buying" such sensationalism, or that a medical doctor considers a disease in terms of marketability, or that cancer is being used for selling. I call B.S., yet it is a classic example of the desire to build a bigger platform through misinformation.

Another example of growing a platform comes from that friend or acquaintance involved in multilevel marketing. Some sell herbal products, while others sell energy drinks, cosmetics, and dietary supplements. "It has transformed my life!" says the friend, who claims the ingredients in her particular product are "proprietary," but really has no idea what she is ingesting or selling. Non-gluten, non-GMO, all-natural...she has no idea what those terms mean. She now labels herself a life and health coach, all designed to build a bigger platform to sell more products while leveraging your esteem need.

If you know a person or company that is trying to grow their following, be on the lookout for bullying.

Esteem: Prestige

My friend, Ellen, describes her fitness instructor's food recommendations: "She knows something I should be eating, so she will tell me about it. She will give me all the arguments as to why she thinks I should be eating it. She will use her position as fitness instructor to influence me as to why she is right, but she will do all this by prefacing it that she is trying to help me and wants what is best for me."

The fitness instructor starts with good intentions, but the bullying begins when Ellen feels judged for not adhering to the fitness instructor's nutrition advice. The instructor is professionally trained in fitness, but not in nutrition. "If this fitness instructor saw me drink a full fat, oh-so-tasty Starbucks drink, I would likely feel guilty and judged after she has preached to me about how bad sugar and caffeine are for me. The same is true if I run into her at a restaurant, and I am enjoying a cheeseburger, because she advises no beef or dairy or gluten" says Ellen.

Again, the fitness instructor wants to help and has implied power, but she is fulfilling a need to build her prestige. Remember bullying often begins where firsthand experience with food production, processing or science ends. If the fitness instructor is not an RDN, food scientist, or a nutrition degree holder, I would suggest you consider her need for prestige before falling prey to bullying, even if it is well-intended. She may be an expert in fitness, but not in eating choices or farming practices.

Are you seeking authority, prestige, affirmation or platform? Be aware that you are more susceptible to food claims that appeal to these motivators. If you believe food choices make you better than someone else, it's time to return to the basics. Have you asked yourself "Is this food nutritious and safe?"

Self-Actualization

I watched my colleague Tammy's food knowledge undergo a radical transformation. Rather than seeing food or certain types of food as the enemy, Tammy, a psychologist and speaker from Louisiana, now believes that food should be viewed as a tool for connection and health.

This was a dramatic change from when we first talked several years ago. Tammy was struggling with infertility and reached out to me for help to sort through the information about food. Tammy and I had a conversation about farming, the truth about food labels, and what really matters in buying food. Her son, now a gleeful kindergartener, is the light of her life, and she recently told me her story. It's a great example of self-actualization in food making informed food choices.

"Over the past couple of years, I've come to see the healing power of food. First, psychologically, there are relationships formed and strengthened over sharing meals together.

"Second, I now believe food is medicine. Previously, I weighed over 200 pounds, had health issues, and was pre-diabetic. By changing my diet, I lost weight and healed my pre-diabetes. I do not eat organic. I eat what's best given my schedule and body (LCHF or low carb high fat).

"My mom is a retired nurse. She always talked about the importance of diet. In many ways, I've been using food to heal since childhood. Specifically, increasing protein consumption to heal following injuries. I started using food to heal more consciously during my years of infertility and researching supplements to increase egg production.

"When I was trying to get pregnant, I looked at the peer reviewed literature and couldn't find any information on food. That's why I contacted you. Your no nonsense, common sense approach resonated with me.

"Most recently, I've elevated food even higher than before. I gained weight due to hormones from fertility treatments and pregnancy." Tammy read journal articles and experimented. She tried exercising five hours/week and taking in 1500 calories/day, then exercised seven hours/week with an intake of 1200 calories/ day. She experimented with different calorie amounts and exercise each week, eventually getting to no exercise and 3,300 calories/ day. Her weight stayed exactly the same in each scenario.

"I was desperate. The calories in/calories out was not working." She ultimately found her answer in LCHF diets with a very pragmatic approach, followed a medical doctor's recommendations, and lost weight while reversing her prediabetes. "While I believe food is amazing and healing, I think people treat it as though it's too precious. I eat what's convenient. I don't have the time nor desire to cook from scratch.

"There is a concept in cognitive psychology called all or nothing thinking. I believe people do this with food. Either they have to be precious with everything, eating organic grapes harvested during a full moon or Oreos washed down with Mountain Dew."

Are we all or nothing? There are many ways to eat; the key is to remember than there's no one solution for everyone; not paleo, vegan, or LCHF. Self-actualization is understanding the science, source, or system well enough to know what works for you. Few people reach the top of the needs hierarchy. Maslow's position is that as people become more self-actualized, they develop wisdom and an understanding of what to do in a variety of situations. In other words, they can sort through information and decide what is best for them.

In my previous two books, I have maintained that it is necessary for people to know the source, science, and system behind food. Self-actualization in eating choices requires a firm grasp of all three of those in order to sort through all of the B.S. claims.

It's a tough level to get to; the science of food is complex, as is the source where it is raised, as is the system in place to protect us. If you find yourself struggling, simplify and—go back to the basics.

Is this food nutritious and safe?

This chapter has looked at how humans are hardwired for survival and the needs that drive us. There's no doubt that our food buying needs, which I believe are closely associated with our most basic psychological needs, can be used by others to bully us. As you measure claims about food, can you get back to the basic question: "Is this food nutritious and safe?" Or, even better, can you eventually rise to the level of self-actualization by better understanding the source, science and system of food? If you find yourself in the middle, where food claims are appealing to your sense of esteem or belonging, remember you are likely being bullied.

Next up, we'll take a look at how and why your brain is being littered with B.S.

CHAPTER 11

Why does it matter to your brain?

One of my favorite ways to relax is to walk on a beach, listening to ocean waves crash while watching for wildlife. I've been fortunate to spend a day as a dolphin trainer, swim with sea turtles, and watch newly hatched turtles make their precarious journey from the beach to the ocean. I love marine life. It pains me to see human litter ruin that beauty and jeopardize wildlife safety.

Yet, I also have to do a gut check when I see consumer environmentalism lead to banning straws in cities like Seattle, corporate statements of elimination of plastic straws by the likes of Disney and Starbucks, and a #stopsucking hashtag after a YouTube video of a sea turtle with a straw lodged in its nose went viral. Why the gut check? Bloomberg News estimates that straws only account for 0.03% by mass of total global plastic waste.

The full story of plastic waste hasn't been told because we are focused on the plastic straw, rather than the big picture of eliminating some of the 275

Mind games are being played to assault your senses and get you to buy Bull Speak.

million metric tons of waste/year.[42] It's a great example of how our desire for belonging can create social change, even though the straw campaign does nothing to reduce our dependence on the four billion plastic bottles used annually. Plastic straws are an easy way for people to feel like they're making a difference, and the campaign to eliminate straws included the right kind of marketing, along with a cool hashtag. It makes us feel good to participate, appealing to our belonging motive, but it doesn't actually solve one of the biggest problems littering the ocean.

What is littering your brain?

It's easier to grab on to the big headlines and believe the latest sensationalized tweet, than to do the gut check and research about the full story. Consequently, our brains may be even more littered than the ocean. This litter can hinder our brains, paralyze our decision-making process, and leave us susceptible to bullying. This chapter will look at why this matters to you, the neuroscience of our food buying decisions and how neuromarketing targets our brains.

Consider our exposure: Pew Research and Hootsuite show these mind-boggling 2018 statistics.

- More adults often get news via social media than printed newspapers, and 71% of Twitter users are reading news there
- Half of all internet users visit YouTube every month, and 70% of those views are mobile
- There are 3.5 billion social media users
- 500 million tweets sent daily
- Two million people pin posts every day, resulting in 100 billion pins on Pinterest
- Instagram users dole out more than 4.2 billion "likes" every day
- 50,000 years of product review videos on YouTube have been watched on mobile devices in the last two years alone,

and Lego has twice as many views as any other brand on YouTube

- Google is the most visited website with 40,000 searches every second. YouTube, which works in 80 languages, is the second most visited site, followed by Facebook

In addition to information overload, our social circle has increased dramatically. We used to have a social circle of about 150 people with whom we could manage relationships. That number has increased to 600 or more people due to social media platforms, according to Barry Wellman at the University of Toronto.[43] I love my friends, but that's a whole lot of people to worry about, don't you think? How do all of these connections and the resulting noise influence the way our brains take in information?

Focusing in a very noisy world

Some studies report that a goldfish has a longer attention span than you or I. Our brains certainly have to work harder today to stay focused. According to Prezi's 2018 State of Attention report, the ability to maintain focus has actually improved over time. However, people have become more selective about the content they consume. A strong narrative or story keeps them engaged and focused, regardless of generation, but narrative is especially important to Millennials.

Advertisers know the power of story and use it to their advantage, especially because consumers may assume advertising mostly tells us about properties of a product. In those stories, advertisers leverage the implied power of product to trigger our esteem and belonging needs.

Are you being conditioned to buy?

One way food marketers leverage needs is through affective conditioning, meaning they take a product and put it next to other things we already feel positively about. For example, an advertising story for baby food may have sunshine, cute babies, and joyful family members as a part of the food's story. These are things we already feel good about, so repeatedly showing the baby food along with the other things we associate with feeling good can make us feel good about the baby food, too. This transfer of feelings from one set of positive associations to another is called affective conditioning.

Associating products with good feelings doesn't just happen in selling products. Affective conditioning is also used by groups to influence your feelings/motives to push their respective platforms. Think about the cute kittens and abandoned puppies featured in the HSUS advertising, asking for your money. Helping these animals makes you feel good about supporting HSUS, though only 1% of their $150 million budget actually goes to kittens and puppies.[44] (As a side note: please do support your local animal shelters.)

A study in *Psychology Today* shows people will pick a product paired with positive items 70-80% of the time, even when they have information that another product is better. The results suggest the most powerful effect of a good advertising story is to create a good feeling about a product by surrounding it with other things you like. Affective conditioning is actually the most effective when you don't realize it's happening.

This study points out why we choose things just because we feel good about them. "The world is a busy place. It is hard for us to feel confident that we have all of the objective facts about anything, whether it is products, people, or choices of things to do. The feelings we have are often a good marker of what is safe to do and what is likely to turn out well. If we have to make a choice, and one of the options just feels good to us, then we are likely to go with the one that feels good."[45]

Do negative associations litter your mind?

Consider the flip side of affective conditioning. What doesn't feel good or comes with negative connotations? Affective conditioning also happens with negative or "absence" associations. A 2017 Fresh Food Shopping Trends survey shows:

1. Nearly half of shoppers define health food by the "absence of the bad stuff."
2. Antibiotic-free chicken sales more than doubled between 2015-2017, going from 12% to 28% of market share.
3. 57% of consumers are motivated by social and cultural factors, specifically less packaging, sustainably produced/grown, organic, animal welfare certified and ecological/biodegradable packaging.

As I've covered extensively in *Food Bullying*, absence claim labels are often Bull Speak. Be sure the story you are buying is real and not littering your brain—or bullying you through feelings associated with esteem and belonging needs.

This is backed up by a different study on our acceptance of chemicals and affective judgements being more strongly related to eating decisions. Intuitive toxicologist Angela Berth, Ph.D., evaluated substances used in consumer products, such as food additives and cleaning additives. There's a lot of misinformation available online about these allegedly dangerous chemicals. The study confirmed consumers have very limited knowledge regarding the processes undertaken to ensure the safety of consumer products—and lack the resources necessary to judge the uncertainty.[46]

Think about the sparkling water flavored with lemon, cayenne, and 19 grams of agave sugar; you can enjoy 16 ounces of La Croix for the low price of around $10. The brand came under fire in a late 2018 lawsuit, when claims were made that testing showed

LaCroix contains a number of artificial ingredients, including linalool, which is also used in cockroach insecticide.[47]

Fire up the fear engines! Associate a high-end beverage with insecticides and chemicals if you want fodder for every level of bullying. Never mind that the chemical can be both naturally and synthetically produced. Or compare different ways in which some chemicals are used, such as sodium as an airplane de-icer or on your dinner table as table salt. Remember, the poison is in the dose. Take chocolate as another example; a huge chocolate bar would likely kill your Chihuahua, but only make your Great Dane sick.

Don't allow negative association to build up your fear. Just because a chemical is used in an insecticide, it doesn't mean it will hurt you. Like with many negative associations, there is often a reasonable, science-based explanation that can reduce or eliminate fear. The poison is in the dose.

The disgust factor

Food mixing together on my plate, strong odors, and bitter tastes disgust me. How about you? Believe it or not, food technologies like gene editing, synthetically produced food additives, or meat created in the lab can evoke feelings of disgust because the new technologies are perceived as unnatural.

I had a hard time grasping that disgust defines food choices, but I also know that the greater the disconnect from our food, the greater the distrust. It makes sense that distrust leads to disgust, but it's important for you to know that reaction is leveraged by bullies. Research has confirmed that disgust about new food technologies reduces one's willingness to eat those foods.[46]

Food bullies leverage this disgust mechanism by trying to turn the debate around new food technologies into a safety discussion, but new food technology acceptance is really about the esteem and belonging needs. Most people are hard-wired for both survival and social acceptance. This brings about thoughts such as, "Will I survive if I eat this new food additive that a tweet said would kill me? Will I be socially ostracized if I buy food that doesn't have the GMO-free label on it?"

There's a lot of science and psychology to wade through, but it boils down to this. People buy what they feel good about, and they don't buy what they are disgusted by. Affective judgements—ethics, cravings, and disgust—are more strongly related to food evaluations and eating decisions. These affective judgements have a far greater impact than the cognitive (reasoned) judgement of food being nutritious and safe. To quote research from Leeds University, "People generally liked and chose to eat foods with high ratings on the positive connotative attributes even if they believed they were not very nutritious, whereas they avoided foods with negative connotative judgements even if they were deemed nutritious and safe to eat."[46]

The mind games of food

Food has become a mind game. Affective conditioning works well to bully us into making quick eating choices because food marketers know we are overwhelmed with information and have precious little time to sort through all the noise. Grocery stores are designed to wage psychological warfare, littering your brain with more than 200,000 messages in one trip around the market.

"Upward of 50% of what we buy in a supermarket we had no intention of buying as we walked in the door," environmental psychologist Paco Underhill says in "The Psychology of the Supermarket." "In the modern 21st-century grocery store, someone has thought through everything in every way, shape, manner or form," Underhill says. "The basic layout hasn't changed much in almost 80 years: I walk in, produce tends to be up front and to the right, meat and seafood tend to be back and to the right, dairy is generally in the back left-hand corner—the deepest section of the store. The reason why is that virtually everyone who walks in has some dairy product on their list."[48]

Supermarkets know what they do best is saturate you with options. 40,000 products in the grocery store means you'd have to use 140 products every day for a year before you could try everything once. That variety is a supermarket's greatest strength—and the biggest threat to shoppers.

Your brain has a hard time saying "no" when it's confronted by thousands of options for breakfast, lunch, and dinner. Have you ever gone grocery shopping for five items and come out with thirty? By appealing to your food buying needs through marketing—and the very design of supermarkets—marketers subtly convince you to spend more time inside. Interestingly enough, grocery stores are like casinos—you're not likely to see clocks, windows, or any indicators of time. The longer you are "trapped" grocery shopping, the more likely products will practically leap in to your cart.

Health halos sell food

As you go through the grocery store, watch for subtle bullying such as the "health-halo effect" and implicit promises that appeal to your motivators. As you're trying to determine which food is a better choice, know that people tend to believe that if one aspect of food is better for you then the entire food must be. For example, if those beloved Cheetos are labeled as high in omegas, are they really healthy? Likely not. Is an organic turkey healthier because it is organic? Likely not.

Cornell University's Food and Brand Lab found that consumers believe organic food has fewer calories and are willing to pay nearly 25% more for it. "Even though these foods were all the same, the "organic" label greatly influenced people's perceptions," they reported. In fact, consumers estimated the organic cookies and yogurt to have significantly fewer calories. Organic is a type of farming, and, based on countless scientific studies, there is no discernable nutritional difference between organically and non-organically produced food. A cookie is still a cookie, no matter what label you slap on it!

Be diligent in guarding your brain against this health halo, knowing labels appeal to your motivators. Likewise, beware of brands implicitly promising you that you'll feel better about yourself (esteem motive) or win praise from friends (belonging motive) when you buy that ethically-harvested coffee or grass-fed steak. Beware of terms like these; they are halo words designed to condition your brain to purchase.

- *All-natural*
- *Clean*
- *_____-free*
- *Farm-raised*
- *Detox*
- *Sustainable*

- *Super food*
- *Local*
- *Ethically-_____*
- *Smart*
- *Cleansing*
- *No toxins*

Sixty-five percent of shoppers indicated they sometimes or always search food labels for "natural" and 58% looked for "clean" in the 2018 MSU Food Literacy and Engagement Poll. I'm sure you're smarter than that. Guard yourself against the marketing overwhelm when you go to the grocery store, or you will fall victim to the bullies who prey on overwhelm.

Assaulting your senses

Have you ever noticed how the cheapest, generic brands are on the lowest shelves? Or that brightly colored, cartoon-adorned boxes are at thigh level for most adults? How about the end of each aisle, known as the endcap, featuring products that are supposedly on sale? Did you notice that you get hungrier after sampling that smoked sausage handed out by the sweet little old lady? Psychological tricks are being played all over the grocery store to assault your senses and get you to buy B.S.

Each of these are marketing tricks to get you to spend more, eat more, and stay longer. That smoked sausage, as well as aromas from the bakery and produce sections, gets your salivary glands working. Once your taste buds are tantalized, your sense of smell leads to less disciplined shopping. The endcap promotions are actually sold to manufacturers to increase sales. They're shortcuts so that we don't have to take the long walk down the grocery aisle. Any parent who has ever shopped with a child can attest to the very real bullying that happens through product placement at the eye level of kids.

As you go through the store, play a game to find food that is the hardest to reach. Your reward will likely be the best priced products. Know that every inch of the grocery store has been meticulously planned, designed, and negotiated to appeal to your needs, either directly or through subtle, psychological means. Don't let your senses be assaulted when buying food, or your brain will become more littered.

The same sensory overload is true in restaurants, even down to the prices on the menus. *Brainfluence* reported that a Cornell study showed that even the way that restaurants display their prices changed how much we spend. They found that menus with simple, spelled-out prices, i.e., those without dollar signs or decimals (e.g. fifteen dollars), resulted in significantly higher spending than $15.00 or "15." If you are in a restaurant where the prices are listed as "twenty dollars" or the like, be aware that they are targeting your brain through neuromarketing.

What does our brain tell us?

All of the bullying strategies I have discussed above are a direct result of a concept called neuromarketing. What is neuromarketing and how is it used to affect our food buying decisions? To understand neuromarketing, you first have to have a basic familiarity with the construction of the brain. The human brain has developed through many years of evolution. The hindbrain controls our basic physiological functions (the bottom two levels of Maslow's hierarchy). It works before the midbrain—primarily our emotion, memory, and motor control functioning (belonging and esteem on the hierarchy) and before our cerebral cortex—our rational brain.

There has been a lot of work done to understand the brain, though it is difficult for most of us to understand the world of neuroscience. The best explanation I've seen is from John Haidt, author of *The Righteous Mind*, who divides the human mind into two parts: an elephant and a rider. The rider is the rational mind—the stream of words and images of which we are fully aware. The elephant is the 99% of the mental processes—the ones that occur outside of awareness but actually govern most of our behavior. For example, the rational mind (the rider), wants a great beach body, but the emotional mind wants those Cheetos. The rational mind (the rider) wants to cook healthier during the cold winter months, but the emotional mind (the elephant) loves the comfort of hearty, rich foods once served by your grandma.

Haidt points out that it becomes the rider's job to serve the elephant. In short, our rational brain often serves our emotional brain. A two-hundred-pound rider isn't likely to move six tons of elephant, unless the rider's brain is more developed than the elephant's brain. This example also points to one of the greatest differences between humans and animals; humans can use our more developed rational brain to corral our emotional brain, just as human intellect allows us to train elephants and other animals.

Food bullies tap into the emotional brain to motivate you to support their platform or product, with little concern about the litter they leave behind. One of the ways to combat this is to know your health, ethical environmental and social standards.

Cleaning up our brain litter

While it may seem very academic, fascinating research is just beginning about how messages around food influence our brains and decision-making. This research can potentially allow us to think rationally, instead of just following the elephant. In order to do that, we have to understand where we're being bullied, which is the focus of Chapter 12.

CHAPTER 12

Where does bullying happen?

One of the most prevalent case studies of misinformation mayhem is the 1998 study from the United Kingdom (U.K.) suggesting a link between common childhood vaccine and autism. This led to considerable fear that has spanned decades, even though the U.K. Department of Health and several other health organizations immediately pointed to the lack of evidence for these claims and urged parents not to reject the vaccine.

Despite this, and media reports that none of the original claims had been substantiated, 20-25% of the public continued to believe in the link between vaccine and autism in 2002. Moreover, 39-53% continued to believe there was equal evidence on both sides of the debate, even with the international campaign to correct the study.

It was then discovered that the author of the study had failed to disclose a significant conflict of interest. He was found guilty of misconduct and lost his

Identify where those with implied power are working to overwhelm your emotional brain and create confusion.

license to practice medicine. The journal officially retracted the article. Yet here we are today with a substantial rise in measles, whooping cough and other preventable diseases that may be directly attributable misinformation now widely disseminated via social media. There's also unnecessary public expenditure on research and public-information campaigns aimed at rectifying the situation. The misinformation surrounding vaccinations prompted some parents to withhold immunization from their children, and, unfortunately, led to a marked increase in vaccine-preventable disease.[49]

Falsely linking vaccinations and autism is a vivid, far-reaching example of misinformation through the implied power of position. Fake news, anyone? If the elephant can drive the rider, it's clear why the emotional brain is where bullies are most likely to target. This is largely done through misinformation, which is rampant in our society today through social media, advertising and even traditional media news reports.

In this chapter, we'll be highlighting those dark places bullies lurk on the food playground, using the implied power of position, platform, and product.

Finding elephants on the playground

Using these three categories of implied power helps make the food bullying playground more approachable than listing every grocery, restaurant, convenience store, and dining room table. Consider the examples listed and where your emotional elephant is likely to be targeted. In other words, where do those with implied power appeal to your emotional brain?

Implied Power	Description	Examples on food playground	Locations
Position	People whose career or expertise gives implied power over others' choices.	Teachers, doctors, nurses, politicians, chefs, fitness instructors, dietitians, farmers	Schools, medical offices, legislature, farms, hospitals, restaurants
Platform	People whose bully pulpit gives them implied power over others.	Friends, celebrities, colleagues, social media connections, journalists, gym nutritionists, activists, parents	Social settings, social media, news, gym, TV, blogs, work, friend groups, family gatherings
Product	Items whose claims, market share, labels give them implied power.	Manufacturers, grocery stores, restaurants, brands marketers, pyramid marketing products, fitness products, supplements	Food labels, menus, health stores, advertisements, social media

Implied power of position

Some of the misinformation having long-term, far-reaching negative consequences may come from sources that aren't as readily identifiable as bullying in medical offices, schools, or restaurants. Some new state and federal regulations are instructive examples. Such is the case in California, where the annual cost for new regulations on citrus growers was shown to be $203 million statewide.[50] Not only do these regulations have significant financial impact on consumers in the grocery store, they also reduce the competitiveness of California farmers. Such far-reaching consequences demonstrate the need for legislators to consider the effect of their actions not only on the buying public, but on the families raising citrus.

The same is true with eggs and a California law passed to change the housing for laying hens. A Cornell University study showed that this law resulted in an increase in egg prices 35 times higher than the overall inflation rate.[51] Higher egg prices may not be a big deal for the average California household, but what about low income families who rely on eggs as an economical source of protein? Looking across the entire U.S. population, the higher egg prices disproportionately harm those with limited means. The argument has also been made that the increase in retail egg prices could cause poorer households to reduce purchase of other essential items such as fruits and vegetables, which also has negative health consequences. Is it fair for the poorest families to bear the consequences of a bad poultry housing law? Shouldn't we be more concerned about the one third of U.S. families that struggle to pay for groceries?

Turning back to the farm, there are several ways to grow food. The same goes for differing dietetic recommendations from RDNs. Both the farmer and the RDN should be expected to follow protocol and be held accountable when they do not. For example, the AND expects dietitians to make science-based recommendations without bias toward organic, GMO, or the like. There is not one right way to farm or eat. Any dietitian or famer who tells you otherwise is a bully.

In the example of vaccination from the beginning of the chapter, the unethical doctor exercised his implied power of position. Bullying with food-related misinformation can happen in a number of locations.

- *Schools*
- *Medical offices*
- *Legislative chambers*
- *Farms*
- *Hospitals*
- *Restaurants*

The implied power of position can be a tough one. Anyone acting as a zealot, judging others or evangelizing that their way is the right way is bullying you through their position. Don't fall for it!

Implied power of platform

The implied power of platform can involve fiction with elements of truth. Consider the *This Is Us* 2018 Super Bowl special. Is it safe to cook in a Crock-Pot? Is your house equipped with fire ladders? Have you replaced the smoke alarm battery? Props to *This Is Us* for bringing fire safety to the forefront, reminding viewers to replace their smoke alarm batteries and have fire ladders. While it's incredibly well-written, it's important to remember that this fictional TV show occurred 20 years ago. Despite providing some good information on fire safety, the show scared people about using crockpots.

Consider the parallel sensationalism motivators used in a popular TV show and farm animal documentaries. Are animals safe on farms? Is it OK to eat meat or consume milk after seeing horrific videos about how one or two bad farmers treat cattle? Have you considered your food ethics? Just as *This Is Us* has created hysteria around slow cookers, some "documentaries" have created hysteria around meat and milk. Written and staged by animal rights activists, the documentaries have great emotional appeal, especially to those who haven't set foot on a farm or ranch.

After all, it's a lot sexier to show the terror of fire or abuse than it is every day, mundane activities. A slow cooker is a rather boring, yet basic, kitchen tool. Caring for animals at 6 a.m. in snow, sun, and sleet is an everyday activity for farmers and ranchers. Both crockpots and animal care can be made more dramatic with sensationalized stories portraying the horrific aftermath of house fires and animals in distress. For example, *This Is Us* didn't focus on the faulty switch that meant the slow cooker should have been put in the trash before it caused a fire. The same is true about "Eating Animals," and other documentaries about the rare abuse on farms, which captures far more attention rather than the everyday management practices of the vast majority of farmers. Both examples of B.S. rely on the implied power of platform to change your established thoughts and buying behavior by appealing to your need for safety.

Implied power of platform can be used for good and bad. Crock-Pot's stock fell immediately after *This Is Us* aired. People dumped their slow cookers in the trash and removed this once-kitchen essential from wedding registries—because of one scene from a fictional show. People have turned away from milk and are questioning their meat choices because they are sickened by the documentaries about farm animals (which are often staged by animal rights activists to change your buying behavior). Because farmers don't have a platform like an award-winning TV show, it's hard to depict what actually happens on farms, particularly when people lack context and are misinformed.

What's a sure sign of implied power of platform? Extreme terms such as industrial agriculture, animal rights, corporate agriculture, environmental poisoning, factory farming, or superiority claims about one type of farming/ranching should put you on high alert.

However, bullying through an implied power platform can also be subtle. If you are an avid follower of a blog, social media group, or TV show, your brain is susceptible to messages designed to engage the emotional elephant instead of the rational rider. Where are you likely to be exposed?

- *Social settings*
- *Blogs*
- *Social media*
- *The gym*

- *Family gatherings*
- *Parent groups*

- *TV*
- *Work*

The power of platform can also happen among those closest to us: our family, friends, and colleagues. While they may not be trying to build a following, they likely have a strong opinion about eating choices and/or want to be seen as an authority. To check this, try asking them "How do you feel about your food?" at your next gathering—as long as you promise not to start a food fight.

Implied power of product

Did you know that Listerine mouthwash falsely claimed the product helped prevent and reduce the severity of colds? This went on for more than 50 years until the U.S. Federal Trade Commission won a legal battle and mandated corrective advertising that withdrew the deceptive claims. In spite of 16 months of advertising that retracted the false, cold-related claims, more than half of Listerine users said that the presumed medicinal effects were a key factor in their purchasing decision.[49] The Listerine example also points to how damaging misinformation can be long-term, as does the vaccine case study.

This is particularly concerning given the misinformation swirling around the food bullying playground about new food technologies like hormones, GMOs, antibiotics, etc. All are topics rife with misinformation. A recent study at Texas Tech showed, through functional MRI imaging, how the brain responds to information about technologies used to produce food, including animal vaccines, hormones, antibiotics, hormone implants, etc.[52] Dr. Davis, a Ph.D. neuroscientist at Texas Tech, conducted the study that compared how our brains process value versus risk.

Upon viewing infographics about each topic, participants perceived the lowest risk and had the most positive attitudes for sustainability and animal welfare compared to their perceptions of specific technologies. The fMRI showed the highest brain activation for antibiotics and hormones, perceived to be the highest risk technologies with the most negative attitudes. We'll get more into exactly where the fMRI shows activation in the brain in later chapters, but there's a whole lot of processing happening right behind your forehead in an area known as the pre-frontal cortex. The medial pre-frontal cortex predicts values-based differences (e.g. sustainability and animal welfare in this study), and the lateral pre-frontal cortex processes factors associated with economic risk, uncertainty, and cognitive control (e.g. antibiotics and hormones).[52]

The study is a fascinating look at how our brains receive and process information (and, potentially, misinformation) about food. There is overlap between the rational and emotional parts of the brain. As we discussed his study by phone, Dr. Davis noted, "It's really never one or the other (emotional or rational); it's always both, but which one wins is the one that's the most engrained or strongest, and that sadly is typically not the rational."

Promoting the implied power of product has been happening for decades across supermarkets, restaurants, convenience stores, and more. Consider this brain research and the food fairytales covered in Section 2 on absence claim labeling, farm size, hormones, and cow farts. Don't let marketing and the implied power of product give strength to your emotional elephant. On the playground of food bullying, you'll see marketing misinformation and product claims, including in:

- *Food labels*
- *Menus*
- *Health stores*
- *Supermarkets*
- *Online retailers*
- *Food advertising*

As discussed in the earlier chapters, our brains don't like too much information. We have about 100 billion neurons, the workers of the brain, processing information. They send messages to each other through billions of connections in coded electrical spikes that travel up to 300 miles per hour. Believe it or not, you have 2.5 miles of neuron networks for every cubic millimeter of gray matter.[53] It's no wonder our brains go a little haywire with all of the information flowing at us.

Research shows that people like to have choices when making a decision but feel less happy about their ultimate decision if they are given too many choices. For example, one consumer study showed that 30% of supermarket customers purchased a jar of jam when offered samples of six different types of jam. But only 3% ended up purchasing a jar when the shoppers were offered 24 different choices.[54]

Translate that to the 40,000 products in a grocery store. Largely driven by Generation X shoppers, private label products (generic) tripled the sales of branded products in 2017. Generics are a key grocery store trend, along with meal kits ($155 million in 2017 retail sales) and online ordering for both home delivery and store pickup.[55] As a harried working mom who lives 20 miles from a supermarket, I can attest to the power of selecting food without ever setting foot in the store! Unfortunately, I also see bullying messages on generic food, meal kits, and online ordering.

Some segments of the population are more prone to being exposed to marketing misinformation. Research shows some restaurants, food and beverage companies specifically target African American, and Hispanic consumers with marketing for their fast-food, candy, sugary drinks, and snacks.[56] This practice raises some questions about unhealthy food marketing aimed at youth under age 18 as a significant contributor to poor diets and diet-related diseases. It stands to reason that Hispanic and Black children and, for that matter, teens in general, who are exposed to this marketing, both in the media and in their communities, will suffer a disproportionate amount of diet-related health problems, including obesity, diabetes, and heart disease.

Food bullying and the implied power of product have long-term consequences reaching well beyond the food playground. Keep that in mind as you look at labels on supplements, consider menu claims, make food choices or shop online. Your risk for exposure to B.S. is high!

The implied power of position, platform, and product can overlap. In some cases, all three can be operating at the same time. For example, a doctor with a national TV or radio show who is pushing her latest diet supplement.

Answering the where

You can be bullied anywhere food is discussed or consumed. Keep the implied power of position, platform, and product in mind—and many places the bullies may lurk on the playground. In so doing, you will be better able to identify where your brain is most susceptible to the bullies. Next, we'll revisit the bullying cycle and when you're most susceptible to it.

CHAPTER 13

When are you the most vulnerable?

A farm mom of a young boy told me this heartbreaking story about how she was bullied when she was pregnant. "Let me share a story that's really hard for me to tell. When I was pregnant with our son, I asked a question that was really important to me, but the doctor's answer is what hurt. This came after he asked me if I wanted to abort my son because he would be born with a cleft lip and palate, which some people just don't want to deal with.

"My question was about what could have caused his cleft lip and palate. The doctor's office staff inquired where I lived, and upon hearing my answer, they told me 'the run-off from the farm fields could have got in the water supply and caused this.' I went home and told my farmer husband.

"I was upset because they assumed it was agriculture's fault. It's not the fault of anyone. It was the way our son was created. God has given me this child, and I'm going to love him and raise him no matter what and not blame

Changing stages in life or diet needs can leave you vulnerable to food bullying.

115

anyone. I'm an adult. I don't blame; I take care of my things." The son is now a ten-year-old 4-H member, who lives a full life, thanks to his mom's willingness to stand up to the doctor's bullying, which I'd say stems from implied power of position.

When are we vulnerable to bullying? During life's most significant changes and challenges, such as finding out your unborn baby is not perfect, moving away to college, becoming a parent, or being diagnosed with a life-altering illness. Change makes us susceptible to thinking more emotionally than rationally. This chapter will revisit the food bullying cycle from Chapter 5 to identify when we are the most vulnerable.

How can the food bullying cycle predict your vulnerability?

Disconnect leads to distrust, which turns into fear. Bullies prey on fear; so the key is to identify fears and stay away from that part of the cycle. As one is bullied more, he becomes more disconnected, and so the cycle continues.

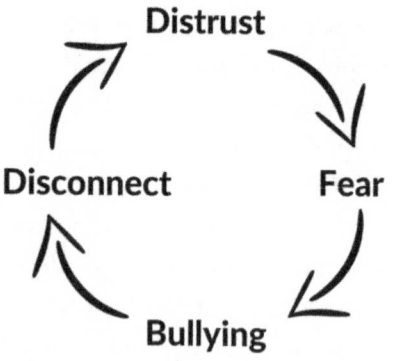

Consider what you do when new information comes in. Do you embrace or question it? What happens in the three pounds of your brain when you learn something new? Those neurons, the workers, start firing thus leaving tracks that deepen as they work together. "Neurons that fire together wire together." In other words, learning actually changes the connection between two neurons—you are creating more connections as you learn more.[57] The question is, what are you learning?

Let's identify when we are the most vulnerable by looking at how this fits with the food bullying cycle—within the context of bullying levels.

Disconnect = vulnerable to zealots, judgers, evangelizers

A college student often feels a disconnect when he is expected to regularly find or prepare food for herself. A dad who just moved to a new neighborhood finds disconnect when he has to go to the grocery store and cannot find his favorite foods. A senior citizen moves to assisted living and has more limited food choices. Each of these examples of disconnect leads to questions about food, an opportunity for neurons to form new connections, and, potentially, gives the elephant of the emotional brain even more power.

Lisa, a marketing professional in Nevada, decided to get fit a few years ago and learn more about what eating choices worked for her body. She found a disconnect with her past eating choices and was then judged and evangelized by people who did not agree with her choice to eat grain-free. "It worked for me. I'd never say that everyone should do that. I got featured in a grain-free site, and a troll went deep into my Facebook and called me out for supporting *Food Truths from Farm to Table*, which has chapters about the value of grains in a healthy diet. I responded that my choices are my choices, and I would never bully someone for his or her choices. I had lots of likes and support after that."

While we are more connected than ever before, it seems we are more disconnected on many levels. Yet brand marketers have more direct access to consumers through social media and work to have consumers become zealots about their products. "Long before Facebook, people have sought to understand what compels people to spread information. A 1966 study by psychologist

Ernest Ditcher identified four reasons why people share brands
with others through word of mouth:

1. Product Involvement: They had such a great experience
   that they had to share it with someone.
2. Self-Involvement: They share with someone to make
   themselves look better, whether to gain attention or to
   show that they are more informed.
3. Other Involvement: They want to share with others to
   help them learn something useful and show they care.
4. Message Involvement: They share because they think it's
   an important or entertaining message.

"Forty-five years after Dichter's study, the New York Times'
Customer Insights Group conducted a new study focusing
specifically on online sharing habits. It turns out, many of the
fundamental reasons people share haven't changed much. What
has changed is how and where they share it."[58]

As you experience disconnect with your food due to changing
stages in life or diet needs, be aware of those who want to convince
you that their way is the only way, or judge your nutrition choices,
or evangelize you to agree with their viewpoint. Don't allow them
to bully you in such ways, or you may end up not trusting your
food. Be particularly vigilant in guarding your brain, especially
when using social media.

Distrust = vulnerable to being evangelized, taunted or shamed

Being a new parent brings more questions than answers—and
so little sleep. You're not really sure you're doing the right thing.
What if you mess up that perfect little human? Other parents can
surely help you with whatever information you need. Warning,
you are vulnerable and on the bullying cycle.

Cami Ryan, a social scientist friend, captured a vivid example of parental food shaming at a community event in Alberta. "There were a number of young moms in the room, balancing cherubic babies on their hips. I eavesdropped on an exchange that went something like this:

> **Mom #1 says proudly:** "Jacob just moved up from rice cereal to baby food."
> **Mom #2:** "Oh, what are you feeding him?"
> **Mom #1:** "Oh, I picked up [Name Brand] baby food at [Store Name]. We are trying that for now. We bought a selection of different vegetables and fruits to see how he likes them."
> **Mom #3:** "Well, I certainly hope that it's organic!"
> **Mom #1:** "Um… I don't know. Well, I don't think so…I…"
> **Mom #2:** "I only feed Kaelynn organic baby food. In fact, I special order it in from [Specialty Baby Food Company]."
> **Mom #3:** "I've heard about that! I feed my baby natural baby food with no preservatives that I get from [Local High-Priced "Natural" Grocery Store].
> **Mom #1:** "But isn't that expensive?"
> **Mom #2:** "Yes, it is more money than the supermarket-bought brands, but my Kaelynn is worth it."
> **Mom #3:** "…After all, the safety and health of our babies is important."
> *awkward silence*
> **Mom #1** looks awkwardly at her feet and shifts healthy, cherubic Jacob to the other hip.
> **Mom #2** and **Mom #3** mentally un-invite **Mom #1** from the next play date."

As Matthew Lieberman says, we are "wired to connect." Our nature is to elevate and preserve status we have within the social "herd." To do so, we need to abide by the collective rules of that social network. If necessary, humans will go to great lengths to protect a position."[59]

Even if you distrust food, it is not something to judge, evangelize or taunt another person about—particularly if there is a little human involved. However, distrust goes well beyond parents. Please know if a person is protecting a "position" about food, your red flag should go up. Food is a personal choice, and the nutrition you select for your family needs to be based on your own social, environmental, nutritional, and ethical standards. Seek information from an expert you can learn to trust before you begin fearing food.

Fear = vulnerable to bullying

At this stage, not only do you feel disconnected from your food and not trust it, you are afraid of it. Let's talk weed killers and carcinogens to highlight how fear can make even the most rational people emotional. Glyphosate kills weeds by targeting a specific pathway and type of bacteria that exists in plants, but not animals or humans.

Many so-called 'watch dog' organizations play the fear card to maximize publicity. That has definitely been the strategy of EWG (an activist group with questionable ethics, discussed in Chapter 9) regarding the most widely-used weed killer. Unfortunately, the strategy has proven successful. Witness, for example, the court case resulted in a $289 million award to a former groundskeeper. It's sad to see this man's condition, but it is also important to note that this court case produced no new scientific data and that juries do not decide science.[60]

The 2015 report by the International Agency Research on Cancer (IARC) classified glyphosate as "probably carcinogenic to humans," after using a narrower base of evidence than other recent, peer-reviewed papers and government reviews from around the world that suggest otherwise. Yet, it's the report most often referred to by those who believe glyphosate causes cancer[61]. By the way, if you're worried about glyphosate causing cancer, you need to know that the same organization also lists bacon and beer are as dangerous as plutonium.

"The European Food Safety Authority looked at 21 human studies and found no evidence for an association between cancer and glyphosate use. The large Agricultural Health Study found no association between cancer and glyphosate in humans. And the 2016 review by Australia's regulator concluded glyphosate was safe if used as directed" according to the American Council on Science and Health.

"The key differences between the IARC's and other reports revolve around the breadth of evidence considered, the weight of human studies, consideration of physiological plausibility and, most importantly, risk assessment. The IARC did not take into account the extent of exposure to glyphosate to establish its association with cancer, while the others did."[61]

Yes, carcinogens sound scary. Yet, everything in your life— including the sun, bacon, and water—have been found to be carcinogenic. Should you be aware? Sure. But when it turns to fearing your food and how that food is produced, you are being bullied. Rely on credible science.

Bullying = running elephant

You are afraid of your food after the unthinkable happened: a family member or friend was diagnosed with cancer. I understand— I've walked in those shoes, caring for a loved one diagnosed with a form of Lymphoma. Earth shattering doesn't quite describe how your world changes, overnight. You begin to fear and question everything. You want to believe anyone who says she has a cure for cancer, because that's better than facing your fears. Be aware that your emotional elephant is running at warp speed during this time of extreme vulnerability and the rational rider is falling off to the side.

The same people who are "selling" a cure for cancer often perpetuate such nutrition myths as "sugar feeds cancer." Cancer Dietitian, Julie Lanford, wants you to know that they are leveraging your fear. She has over a decade of experience in oncology and writes, "every cell in the body requires glucose for fuel, including cancer cells. We get glucose from all carbohydrate foods. If we don't eat enough carbohydrates, the cells (normal and cancer) still demand a source of glucose, and the body makes it by breaking down protein from our muscles and immune system. In order to minimize muscle loss and immune compromise, we need to provide a consistent source of carbohydrates through the diet whenever possible.

"Cells use glucose the way cars use gas. With normal driving, our car uses varying amounts of gas depending on whether we are idling or accelerating. Normal cells divide at varying rates, some every three days and some every three months, or more. During cell division, more glucose is used, much like an accelerating car uses more gas. But after cell division, it returns to more of an idling state, using less glucose.

"Cancer cells are like cars with the accelerator stuck to the floor, using glucose at high rates, because they are dividing at much faster rates than normal cells. If you still want to be able to drive your car, you cannot fix it if it has the accelerator stuck down simply by letting it run out of gas. For the same reason, you cannot starve cancer cells of glucose because you will also be depriving your healthy cells of fuel. The cancer cells are much more tenacious than the normal ones and will persist at the expense of the rest of the body."[62]

Whether it's cancer and sugar or other nutrition claims, know that claims feeding into fear are very unhealthy. They send your elephant running astray, looking for anything else that appeals to your emotional brain! Fear is a real emotion that leaves you vulnerable especially during life's most challenging times. Recognize your fear, stand up to the bullies, and rely on credible experts to break the bullying cycle.

Check your buying behavior

Bottom line, use the bullying cycle as a tool to check when you are most vulnerable. Keep in mind that it is an ongoing cycle, and that you will experience the different levels of bullying at different times. In the next chapter, we'll address how to stand up to those bullies, the final step in developing your own food story.

CHAPTER 14

How do you stand up to bullies?

Food bullying isn't just an American problem. In Germany, Agnes and her parents created a Facebook page called "Ferienhof Greggersen" (Greggersen Farm) for their prospective vacationers and people interesting in farming. They wanted to showcase their dairy farm and connect with people outside of agriculture. However, they got more than they bargained for when Agnes posted a video with a child drinking a glass of milk. The vegans came out in full force to comment on the video, calling their activism a "vegan shitstorm." Among other vicious, repulsive statements, the vegan bullies actually suggested the family should die. Agnes didn't know what happened, so she removed the video and made the page invisible. Turns out that was the first of many "vegan shitstorms" on Facebook pages of German farmers.

Agnes then reported they made a video with their farm organization to show others what happened to them. "We knew we wouldn't reach the bad vegans, *Be aware of how you process information and work to keep your brain focused on rational decisions.*

but we wanted to reach regular people and help other farmers not be afraid of sharing their story in social media. We turned the negative bullying experience into a positive experience and generated more results. It's clear these vegans want to spread their opinion and don't want to have the farm side in social media." Agnes said it's her motivation to help people understand by telling stories from the farm side of the food plate. Unfortunately, more and more farmers are finding themselves under personal attack. In the U.S., less than 1.5% of the population is on a farm or ranch.

Dealing with bullies is hard. Cutting through all of the B.S. on the food bullying playground is hard. And knowing what your own brain is supposed to be doing is hard. Then again, most things worth doing are hard. This chapter will explore how to build your own food story, which will better equip your rational brain to stand up to the bullies.

Know your brain

Did you know your brain "lights up" when processing information? A great cut of steak makes your brain light up like a Christmas tree because of increased reward connectivity, shown in images from fMRI.[63] Modern technology has allowed the healthy brain to be studied only for the last 25 years, and fMRI is a critical tool in conducting that research. When I interviewed Dr. Davis from Texas Tech, he talked about how neuroscience is "a window into how the brain works to help us improve human decision making." He sees this type of research as an opportunity to devise strategies to think rationally and improve decision-making. His recent study used brain images to measure the response of consumer perceptions about animal welfare technologies.[64]

In order to understand how information is processed, it's important to look at where the brain processes it. According to Davis, we have to open up the hood and understand what's actually happening. The prefrontal cortex (PFC), located behind our forehead, is where explicit attitudes and decisions come from. The PFC, which is far more highly developed in humans than any other species, contains two parts:

1. **Lateral PFC:** In simple terms, it tracks how much you are working to process things and sort out conflicting information. The lateral PFC region sorts out all of the different pieces of information to control intellectually and determines how we are focusing on that information to influence behavior. It predicts economic risk and uncertainty processing. In the Texas Tech study, the lateral PFC area was more highly activated for the "riskier" food technologies such as hormones and GMOs. This heightened activation, may be related to having to sort out the conflicting signals from our "automatic emotional" response to not trusting technologies and the more rational information. In a sense, this brain region is the rational part, and what it decides to do is based largely on sorting out all of the competing information.

2. **Medial PFC:** It tracks how much you like things. The medial PFC is much more tied to value-based processing and is part of what would be considered the emotional component of the brain. It tends to track what people are subjectively valuing. The fMRI shows more activity if you like the information or are more confident about your choice. In the Texas Tech study, the medial PFC held positive attitudes toward information about animal vaccines and animal welfare. However, medial PFC activity it is not purely emotional because it is also sensitive to intellectual information. The medial PFC is the brain region that's involved with subjective valuations; it blends both emotional and rational information to get to decisions.

What does all of this brain work mean to you? In the ideal world, the rational rider would control the emotional elephant when receiving and processing new information about food. But you and I don't live in an ideal world, and often the emotional elephant prevails. What we can do? First, become better aware of the way the brain processes information, and then work to keep our brains wired toward rational decisions. This is particularly important when receiving new information. If your brain is overwhelmed, it will default emotional decision-making, leaving you susceptible to bullying.

People often hold a natural dislike of food technology and higher perceptions of associated risk. It's also proven that we don't like too much information and our brains become overwhelmed with the many claims that leverage our food buying needs. Do you find yourself questioning food because of the information littering your brain? Are your choices overwhelming?

Set boundaries

Bullies are only as powerful as we allow them to be. So, how can we work to better mobilize our rational brain to overcome food-related bullying? A leading authority suggested, *in Psychology Today*, the following steps to take when dealing with bullying.[65] I've added concrete examples (in italics) about how I set boundaries when selecting food at restaurants, online, and in grocery stores.

1. Be confident. Remember that bullies prey on fear. *When a food claim scares me, I turn away from the food. I find a farmer, food scientist or RDN to clarify any confusing claim.*
2. Stay connected. Bullies make their victims feel disconnected, but they're actually seeking attention. *Keep a close circle, find experts whom you can question and call on as needed. Remember, it's impossible for any one of us to know everything there is about food, but collectively we have power.*

3. <u>Look for simple, unemotional language.</u> *I often shop at Aldi's or online because the labels are simpler. There are fewer choices, and I don't have to filter through emotional brand claims. If at a supermarket, I select store brands (unless we've had a bad experience with a certain food) and turn away from marketing on food packages or in the aisles.*

4. <u>Set limits.</u> *I refuse to spend more than a 30 or 60-minute chunk of time in the grocery store and will limit the number of choices I have to make. I also "turn off" my emotional elephant as much as I can and find moving fast keeps the rational rider more in control.*

5. <u>Act quickly and consistently.</u> *I do not frequent restaurants that make clean-eating claims, have food safety concerns, or evangelize their way as the only way. I also discard information that is not scientifically-based when filtering social media and rely on those with firsthand expertise, such as farmers and dietitians.*

6. <u>Strike when the iron is cold.</u> *Rather than responding to pressures of the moment from peer groups, or social media trolls, and share my platform (meeting several of their needs on Maslow's hierarchy), I wait to respond to claims with a cooler head than the bully. I only respond to benefit those that are watching and interested in learning.*

Control your own story

Ninety-five percent of Americans report that they look for healthy options when food shopping, based on a study conducted by the International Food Information Council and American Heart Association. They are most likely to consult food labels for healthfulness information when buying a product for the first time. However, only 28% say it's easy to find healthy foods.[66]

Why so? Likely, in large part, because of the plethora of food claims. And what is healthy, anyhow? It's important for you to identify your own standards to arm yourself against the bullies discussed throughout this book. I'll talk more about identifying those four standards in Chapter 20, but it's essential to control your food story.

After 18 years of working to build connections between farm and food, I have identified six basic building blocks of a story allow us to act quickly and frame information in a way our brains can rationally process. As you consider your own food story, I would challenge you to consider these questions.

1. **Who is likely to bully you?** Remember to step back and ask yourself which bullying level they fall into: zealot, judge, evangelist, taunter, or shamer. Also ask which implied power the bully in questions is leveraging to influence you: position, platform, or product?

2. **What are their motivators?** Be on the lookout for messages about eating choices that leverage your needs for esteem (tradition, altruism, and activism) and belonging (prestige, affirmation, authority, platform). Return to the basic question: is this food nutritious and safe?

3. **Why does it matter to you?** Guard your brain against information overload, affective conditioning (positive and negative), and other psychological warfare. What are your own health, ethical, environmental, and social standards?

4. **Where are you likely to be bullied?** The playground of food bullying reaches anywhere food is discussed or consumed, including doctors' offices, classrooms, dinner tables, etc. But remember the implied power of position, platform, and product to help identify locations where you're likely to be bullied.

5. **When are you the most vulnerable?** Keep the food bullying cycle in mind. Disconnect leads to distrust, which turns into fear. Bullies prey on fear, so the key is to identify

fears and stay away from that part of the cycle. Life changes and challenges leave you especially susceptible.

6. **How can you stand up to bullying?** Keep your emotional elephant in check and employ strategies that empower your rational brain when you've identified food bullying. Set boundaries by using an action plan.

Developing your food story

Congratulations, you made it through the information-intense Section 3. It has intended to give you background on food bullying and strategies to help you develop your own story. This section has outlined the players on the food bullying playground, their motivators, how our brains are being targeted, where bullying is likely to happen, when you're the most vulnerable, and how to stand up to the bullies. My goal in these six chapters was to provide you with examples and ideas to help you avoid buying B.S.

Moving on to Section 4, I will try and illuminate much of the misunderstanding and complexity surrounding the subject of food labels and offer evaluation tools you can use to sort the meaningful and measurable labels from the B.S.

SECTION 4

Thinking through B.S. to overcome bullying

CHAPTER 15

Defining food labels & looking for B.S.

"Pan fry slowly on low-medium heat until bacon renders and is cooked to your desired crispness. If you don't know how to cook bacon, please contact your elected officials and complain about our education system. Every American should know how to cook bacon. Seriously." Such are the cooking instructions on the back of a package Black River Meats bacon.

After a picture of the bacon directions received several thousand likes on Facebook, I verified it on Snopes and found that the brand marketers did this as a "mixture of humor and seriousness, because what's the world coming to if people don't know how to cook something as simple as bacon?" The meat company also thought they "could better promote safety awareness if they could get people to step back and relax a little by leavening their packaging with some humor to break the tension" in the contentious food arena.[67]

What a great idea! If more food packages offered humor to break the tension, perhaps we wouldn't have to worry about

Know which food labels have measurement and meaning; disregard B.S. labels.

food bullying. Yet, it's clear that labels are often dictating our eating choices, whether purchasing groceries or dining at a restaurant. Let's look at which labels are meaningful and those that you can filter out as B.S.

What are B.S. labels?

"It's notable that the most popular terms consumers search for on food labels are also the most ambiguous," said Sheril Kirshenbaum, co-director of the MSU Food Literacy and Engagement Poll. "Natural doesn't necessarily imply something is healthy. For example, arsenic occurs naturally, but we shouldn't eat it."[68]

Keep in mind that there are two types of labels: those mandated by FDA, presumably science-based, and manufacturer marketing labels that frequently target your need for esteem or belonging. Ask yourself if a label claim lack definitive measurement or meaning? In other words, are you worrying about a label because of something you read on social media? Is it a topic du jour or a concern of a friend? Or, is there a definitive, verifiable difference in the food, such as the Nutrition Facts Label?

Let me make it simple. Below are examples of label claims that aren't regulated; they are pure marketing and lack measurement and meaning. They are B.S.!

- Clean
- Local
- Family farm
- Non-GMO
- All-natural
- Superfood
- Healthful
- _____-free

- Ethically-_____
- Farm-raised
- Smart
- Detox
- Whole
- Cleansing
- Transparent
- Sustainable

See how much simpler it is if you just trash the useless labels? Filter them out immediately, and move on to labels with definitive meanings, or turn to the Nutrition Facts Label.

Which labels are FDA monitored and measured?

Health claims are regulated by the Food and Drug Administration (FDA) and include any claim on a food label, including a dietary supplement, that implies, expresses, or shows a relationship exists between "the presence or level of substance in the food and a disease or health-related condition." These claims are limited to those about disease reduction and cannot be claims about the diagnosis, cure, mitigation, or treatment of disease.[69]

Going through nearly 500 pages of FDA, USDA and Food Safety Inspection Service (FSIS) food labeling documents makes me want to bang my head against a cement wall. It is crazily complicated, but I've done my best to filter out examples of label claims that are measurable, monitored, and science-based. You can find a compilation of resources detailing label claims at http://causematters.com/foodbullying/info.

Genetics

- **Bioengineered (BE):** A new label will designate any product with bioengineered crops, by 2022. BE does not convey any information about the health, safety, or environmental attributes of bioengineered food as compared to non-bioengineered counterparts. A this point in time, you won't see any bioengineered meat or milk products, as it has not been approved. Bioengineering is a precise science that allows a more refined outcome than traditional breeding: taking one gene (a small part of DNA) from one plant and placing it another. Contrary to rumors, approved biotechnology uses naturally occurring genes and is heavily researched and regulated. For example, companies invest around $150 million and 15 years in research before biotechnology seeds are approved—far more than any "regular" seed. USDA's definition is "a food that contains genetic material that has been modified through invitro rDNA techniques and for which the modification could not otherwise be obtained through conventional breeding or found in nature."

Production System

- **Conventional:** Common term for modern farming practices, but also used to describe a farm that is not certified organic. Conventional farms can be small or large, adapting a wide variety of practices and technologies. Some are Community Supported Agriculture (CSA) farmers, others farm thousands of acres. Size does not define the farm, family does.

- **Organic:** Certified organic must be verified by a third party, as mandated by the USDA marketing standards. The USDA Organic label is the only certified federal program so look for that seal if you want organics. USDA defines organic as "a labeling term that indicates that the food or other agricultural product has been produced through approved methods."
  - 100% organic=all the ingredients in the food are organic.
  - Organic=at least 95% of the ingredients are organic.
  - Made with organic ingredients=at least 70% of the item is organic.

Calories

- **Low-calorie:** 40 calories or less per serving.

- **Reduced-calorie:** At least 25% fewer calories per serving compared with the full calorie version of the food.
- **Light or lite:** Half as much fat (or even less) than a similar food. If the food gets less than half its calories from fat, "light" or "lite" means it has half as much fat as a similar food or 30% fewer calories.

Sugars

- **Sugar-free:** Less than ½ gram of sugar per serving.
- **Reduced sugar:** At least 25% less sugar per serving compared with the regular-sugar food.
- **A note on sugars:** A sweetener is a sweetener, no matter the label you slap on it. Agave and High Fructose Corn Syrup (HFCS) are both caloric equivalents to sugar, which is harvested from sugar cane or beets. HFCS has come under a firestorm for the commercial use of it as a sweetener. It's a by-product of wet milling corn and meets the FDA requirements for the use of the term 'natural.'

Fats

- **Fat-free:** Less than ½ gram of fat per serving.
- **Low-fat:** 3 grams of fat or less per serving.
- **Reduced-fat:** At least 25% less fat when compared with the regular-fat version of the food.

Sodium

- **Low-sodium:** Food with 140 mg. or less of sodium per serving.
- **Very low-sodium:** 35 mg. or less of sodium per serving.
- **Reduced or less salt or sodium:** 25% less than a similar food.
- **Light in sodium or lightly salted:** Less than 50% salt or sodium than a similar product.

Other Health Claims

- **Heart-Check Certification:** The product must meet specific nutrition requirements. The Heart-Check program has seven different categories of certification, and each category has a different set of nutrition requirements. All products must also meet government regulatory requirements for making a coronary heart disease health claim. There are additional requirements for specific food categories.[70]
  - o Total Fat: Less than 6.5 grams.
  - o Saturated Fat: 1 gram or less and 15% or less calories from saturated fat.
  - o Trans Fat: Less than 0.5 grams (also per label serving). Products containing partially hydrogenated oils are not eligible for certification.
  - o Cholesterol: 20 mg. or less.
  - o Sodium: One of four sodium limits applies depending on the particular food category: up to 140 mg., 240 mg., or 360 mg. per label serving, or 480 mg. per label serving and per amounts typically consumed. See Sodium Limits by Category for details.
  - o Beneficial Nutrients (naturally occurring): 10% or more of the Daily Value of 1 of 6 nutrients (vitamin A, vitamin C, iron, calcium, protein or dietary fiber).
- **Whole Grain Stamp:** There are three different varieties of the Whole Grain Stamp, reflecting different amounts of whole grains, a valuable source of fiber:[71]
  - o 100% Stamp: All of a product's grain ingredients are whole grain. There is a minimum requirement of 16 grams—a full serving—of whole grain per labeled serving.

o 50%+ Stamp: At least half of the product's grain ingredients are whole grain. There is a minimum requirement of 8 grams—a half serving—of whole grain per labeled serving.

o Basic Stamp: Product contains at least 8 grams—a half serving—of whole grain, but may contain more refined grain than whole.

If you're looking for the latest information, check https:// causematters.com/foodbullying/info for links to labeling information from FDA and USDA. It complex and complicated with hundreds of pages of documents, so I've only covered the basics here as a quick reference.

No B.S. labels

Bull Speak does not belong on labels. Turn away from the food or organization making B.S. claims. In the next chapter, I'll help you evaluate labels on the food buying needs hierarchy.

CHAPTER 16

Evaluating food claims

Have you ever dreamed of looking like Tom Brady or his model wife, Gisele? A case study in building a platform, the Brady's personal chef, Allen Campbell, shared the details of the diet he "designed" for the couple before he left. It's plant-based, organic, gluten-free, GMO-free, sugar-free, fungus-free, caffeine-free, salt-free, and dairy free.

"Campbell has managed to fit in every single piece of dietary insanity on the planet into one meal plan," notes Yvette determent, also known as SciBabe.[72] "It's borderline impressive how someone can cram so much non-scientifically based information, fear-mongering of healthy foods, and just plain old bullshit into one neatly tied, organically wrapped package. Yes, the diet may sound healthy, given that it's loaded up on fruits and vegetables. But it also cuts out so much food that it's composed of more air than fiber." Her piece is a rather humorous look at the chef's food claims, though you'll have to pardon the language. This chapter will explore a few more of the claims made on the playground of food bullying and provide strategies on how to evaluate them.

Go back to the basics and ask "Is this food nutritious and safe?"

FDA on false and misleading label claims

It's not just celebrities and chefs making questionable food claims; it's also food companies. Clear back in 2010, FDA's Commissioner of Food and Drugs at the time, Dr. Margaret A. Hamburg, sent a letter to food manufacturers about the need for a more understandable front-of-package labeling system and the number of label claims that may be false or misleading. "To address these concerns, FDA is notifying a number of manufacturers that their labels are in violation of the law and subject to legal proceedings to remove misbranded products from the marketplace. While the warning letters that convey our regulatory intentions do not attempt to cover all products with violative labels, they do cover a range of concerns about how false or misleading labels can undermine the intention of Congress to provide consumers with labeling information that enables consumers to make informed and healthy food choices. For example:

- Nutrient content claims that FDA has authorized for use on foods for adults are not permitted on foods for children under two. Such claims are highly inappropriate when they appear on food for infants and toddlers because it is well known that the nutritional needs of the very young are different than those of adults.

- Claims that a product is free of trans fats, which imply that the product is a better choice than products without the claim, can be misleading when a product is high in saturated fat, and especially so when the claim is not accompanied by the required statement referring consumers to the more complete information on the Nutrition Facts Label.

- Products that claim to treat or mitigate disease are considered to be drugs and must meet the regulatory requirements for drugs, including the requirement to prove that the product is safe and effective for its intended use.

- Misleading "healthy" claims continue to appear on foods that do not meet the long- and well-established definition for use of that term.
- Juice products that mislead consumers into believing they consist entirely of a single juice are still on the market. Despite numerous admonitions from FDA over the years, we continue to see juice blends being inaccurately labeled as single-juice products."[73]

I realize that not everyone trusts the government and there have been concerns around food companies unduly influencing FDA, but I also believe this is the system that best protects our food. I do believe government agencies should be even more aggressive in regulating food labels, given the infractions that have been cited over the decades. Nonetheless, the black and white "panel" known as the Nutrition Facts Label is a reliable place to look for truth.

Put labels on the food buying needs hierarchy

Nearly a decade after the FDA warning letter, the food bullying has intensified. New labels are slapped on foods in an effort to appeal to our belonging and esteem needs, while companies try to sell more food. Consider some of the B.S. labels from Chapter 15 and where they fit on the food buying needs hierarchy on the following page. Are there others you'd place in these boxes? Those are the labels you can quickly dismiss to simplify your food buying.

FOOD BUYING NEEDS

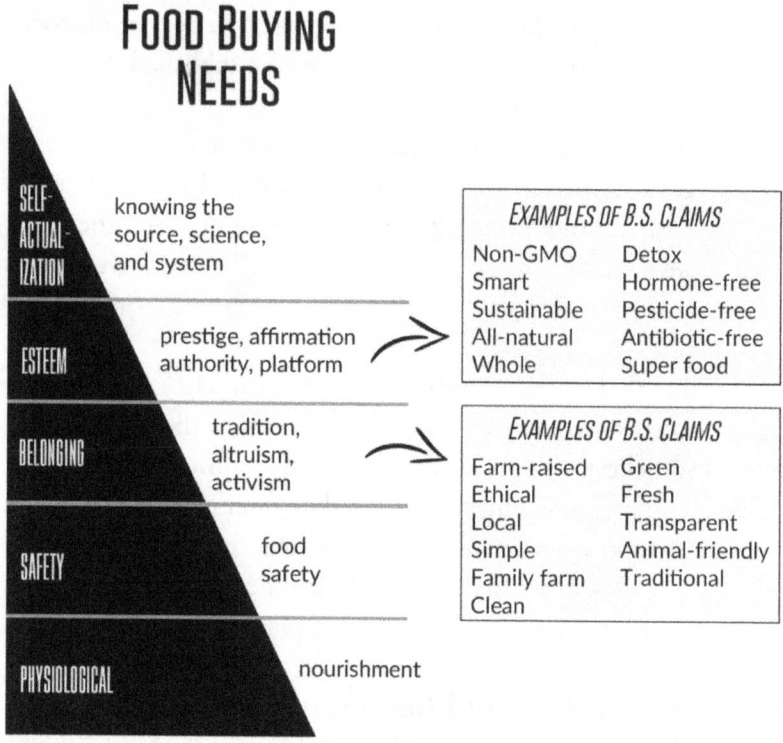

SELF-ACTUALIZATION	knowing the source, science, and system
ESTEEM	prestige, affirmation authority, platform
BELONGING	tradition, altruism, activism
SAFETY	food safety
PHYSIOLOGICAL	nourishment

EXAMPLES OF B.S. CLAIMS

Non-GMO	Detox
Smart	Hormone-free
Sustainable	Pesticide-free
All-natural	Antibiotic-free
Whole	Super food

EXAMPLES OF B.S. CLAIMS

Farm-raised	Green
Ethical	Fresh
Local	Transparent
Simple	Animal-friendly
Family farm	Traditional
Clean	

Did you know that most Americans eat and drink a third of their calories away from home? Since we consume nearly twice as many calories away from home now as we did in the 1970s, the FDA also started requiring restaurants or grocery stores with more than 20 locations to list calorie information.[74] Hopefully this will help you to make healthier, better-informed meal choices rather than having to rely on the B.S. claims often made by restaurants.

Is this food nutritious? Understand the Nutrition Facts Label

It is the most the functional label on food, though it lacks flash. The Nutrition Facts Label is the best reference point on a food package to avoid B.S. All manufacturers are required to use the new Nutrition Facts Label before 2021.[75] Serving sizes and daily values are updated, along with emphasizing calories, listing actual amounts of nutrients, and detailing added sugars. You can see an example of the Nutrition Facts Label, with the changes approved in 2018, below.

NUTRITION FACTS LABEL
YOUR BEST GUIDE TO AVOID B.S.

	Nutrition Facts	
Servings: — larger, bolder type	8 servings per container **Serving size** **2/3 cup (55g)**	— Serving sizes updated
	Amount per serving **Calories** **230**	— Calories: larger type
	% Daily Value*	
	Total Fat 8g **10%**	
	Saturated Fat 1g **5%**	
	Trans Fat 0g	— Updated daily values
	Cholesterol 0mg **0%**	
	Sodium 160mg **7%**	
	Total Carbohydrate 37g **13%**	
	Dietary Fiber 4g **14%**	
New: added sugars —	Total Sugars 12g	
	Includes 10g Added Sugars **20%**	
	Protein 3g	
Change in nutrients required	Vitamin D 2mcg 10%	— Actual amounts declared
	Calcium 260mg 20%	
	Iron 8mg 45%	
	Potassium 240mg 6%	
	* The % Daily Value (DV) tells you how much a nutrient in a serving of food contributes to a daily diet. 2,000 calories a day is used for general nutrition advice.	— New footnote

This box of information, from FDA, is the single best place to go for sound data on a food package. Flip your food package to find it and ignore other claims if you want science-based facts. Use the Nutrition Facts Label as your "go-to" when determining the nutritional value of food. It's really that simple.

If you're in a hurry, key highlights can often be found on a "Facts Up Front" label on the front of package. Fast facts include number of calories, fat, and sodium content, added sugars, daily values, etc. As long as you are looking at the box with the facts taken directly from the Nutrition Facts Label, the Facts Up Front Label is a great quick reference.

Next, we'll take a look at how to answer questions about food safety. Unfortunately, it's not as simple as reading one label.

Is this food safe? Allergens

Food can kill, especially if you suffer from food allergies. Knowing allergens is a food safety imperative for the 32 million Americans with food allergies. More than 160 foods have been identified to trigger food allergies in sensitive individuals, but there are eight major food allergens that account for 90% of all food allergies. The Food Allergen Labeling and Consumer Protection Act of 2004 requires that food labels must clearly identify the food source names of any ingredients that are one of the eight major food allergens or contain any protein derived from a major food allergen (e.g. contains wheat, milk, and soy). The eight are:[76]

- *milk*
- *egg*
- *fish*
- *crustacean shellfish*

- *tree nuts*
- *wheat*
- *peanuts*
- *soybeans*

Look for the allergens to be clearly labeled, "may contain…," and check the ingredient list to be sure of the safety of your food if you are concerned about allergies.

Is this food safe? Ingredients list

How many times have you flipped a food product over to inspect the ingredients? Some of the terms may scare you, but know this is a federally regulated list. FDA requires manufacturers to use the common ingredient name unless there is a regulation that provides for a different term. The order the ingredients are listed is determined by descending order of weight, starting with the ingredient that weighs the most.

Keep in mind that some products are listed by their scientific name. Contrary to claims by celebrity food bullies, the benefit of an ingredient listing is not determined by your ability to pronounce it. Dihydrogen monoxide sounds scary, but it is an essential ingredient to life that you consume multiple times each day. Remember the ingredients from eggs and blueberries? It's OK to eat what you can't pronounce and chemicals are naturally a part of foods.

Is this food safe? Food date labels

Another safety concern is eating food before it goes "bad." But how is bad defined? We waste $161 billion or 40% of our food annually. Some of this comes from the rotten vegetable 'science experiment' at the back of your refrigerator, some food waste is from those selling food, and some of it comes from our confusion over food expiration dates.

A recent national online survey showed that consumers frequently misunderstood food date labels such as "best before" and "sell by." More than one-third of respondents incorrectly thought these date labels were federally regulated, and 26% were unsure. They reported discarding food based on label dates with significantly more frequency than other consumers.[77] The research found that 84% discarded food near the package date "at least occasionally," and 37% reported that they "always" or "usually" discard food near the package date.

Aside from food recalls and visual/odor appraisal (is there mold on the produce, does the meat look right, how does it smell, etc.), it's pretty clear that food expiration dates are a key food safety evaluation tool in the U.S. These dates are largely unregulated, although new voluntary standards are coming into effect. Communication about dates is needed as this research about food date labels found widespread confusion, leading to unnecessary discards, increased waste, and food safety risks.

Raw chicken was most frequently thrown out because of the food date label. 69% report they "always" or "most of the time" discard by the listed date. 62% reported discards of prepared foods by the date label, and 61% reported discards of deli meats. Soft cheeses were near the bottom of the list. Only 49% said they discarded by the date label, followed by 47% throwing out canned goods and breakfast cereals.

Prepared foods, deli meats, and soft cheeses are particularly at risk of contamination from listeria, a bacteria which grows quickly in refrigerated conditions. Despite concerns of listeria, soft cheeses were rarely discarded by the labeled date. On the other hand, raw chicken was frequently discarded even though it would be cooked prior to consuming and is not considered as big a risk.[77]

Keep in mind that bacteria, dirt, and germs happen. Keep your meat safe by using a thermometer to check that your meat is always cooked to the recommended minimum temperatures: roasts and steaks to 145°F, poultry to 165°F, ground meat to 160°F, and fish to 145°F. Check http://fightbac.org for other great food safety tips.

Your take away? Don't trash food just because of a date on the package; use your nose and eyes to detect food spoilage, then cook it properly to be sure it's safe. FDA reports that "Manufacturers provide dating to help consumers and retailers decide when food is of best quality. Except for infant formula, dates are not an indicator of the product's safety and are not required by Federal law."

The USDA goes on to say that "to reduce consumer confusion and wasted food, FSIS recommends that food manufacturers and retailers that apply product dating use a 'Best if Used By' date. Research shows that this phrase conveys to consumers that the product will be of best quality if used by the calendar date shown.

Foods not exhibiting signs of spoilage should be wholesome and may be sold, purchased, consumed, and even donated beyond the labeled 'Best if Used By' date."[78]

Is this food safe? Processing codes

You can check the manufacturing date yourself if you know how to read the codes on food packages. The first thing to understand is that most processors use Julian dating, representing consecutive days of the year. This means January 1 is 001 and December 31 is 365. It also helps to know that most food companies start their manufacturing year in June and begin their coding with the letter A. That means that A is June, B is July, etc.

The good news is that all packages of food have codes that you can use for tracing where and when your food was processed. For example, all containers of meat, poultry, and egg products must be labeled with a USDA mark of inspection and establishment, which is assigned to the plant where the product was produced and can be found with a P or EST on the USDA seal. The bad news is that these codes are regulated by different agencies, so you may have to check a few different places depending what food you're buying. However, with a little detective work, you can trace your food.

- Eggs: All USDA Grade A eggs show the packing date right after the processing plant number at the end of the carton
- Meat & Poultry: Download USDA's MPI (Meat & Poultry Inspection Services) app
- Milk: Use Where is My Milk From (https://whereismymilkfrom.com/finding-my-code)
- Other foods: Visit Code of Federal Regulations (https://ecfr.gov) for the specific food

How do you handle all of this information?

Yes, there are a lot of details to take in, but keep your own important role top-of-mind. Your practices are the best way to keep your food safe; food handling, cooking, and storage are essential to preventing foodborne illness. Remember that you won't see or taste the harmful bacteria that cause illness. FSIS recommends the four steps of the Food Safe Families campaign to help keep food safe.[79]

- **Clean:** Wash hands and surfaces often.
- **Separate:** Don't cross-contaminate.
- **Cook:** Cook to the right temperature.
- **Chill:** Refrigerate promptly.

The purpose of the last two chapters has been to help you locate, understand, and interpret science-based information that can be found either on food packaging or from credible sources. If you are armed with this reliable information about the food you buy and consume, you can protect yourself from bogus marketing claims, biased reporting, misinformation from friends, and other sources of Bull Speak.

In the final chapter of Section 4, we'll take a look at how to best manage the noise on the chaotic food playground.

CHAPTER 17

Managing information literacy

If Listerine doesn't cure colds, weenie water doesn't prevent aging, and vaccines don't cause autism, then why do smart people still believe these to be true? Never before in human history has so much information been available. Likewise, never has so much misinformation been so readily accessible.

"If a majority believes in something that is factually incorrect, the misinformation may form the basis for political and societal decisions that run counter to a society's best interest. If individuals are misinformed, they may likewise make decisions for themselves and their families that are not in their best interest and can have serious consequences.

"For example, following the unsubstantiated claims of a vaccination-autism link, many parents decided not to immunize their children, which has had dire consequences for both individuals and societies, including a marked increase in vaccine-preventable disease and hence preventable hospitalizations, deaths, and the unnecessary expenditure of large

Develop the skills to locate, evaluate, and effectively use food information.

amounts of money for follow-up research and public-information campaigns aimed at rectifying the situation." This from the authors of the "Misinformation & Its Correction" paper.[80]

It's clear that the food bullying playground is filled with half-truths and misinformation. Therefore, it's critical we equip ourselves to better manage information, filter out the B.S., and clear the litter from our brains in order to make rational decisions. This chapter will focus on the importance of information literacy in being able to research and understand the issues related food bullying.

Why information literacy?

My friend Eliz went to high school orientation last fall, in preparation for her twin daughters' senior year. She noticed many teachers were talking different kinds of literacy: statistics was referred to as data literacy and English was about information literacy—which included evaluating sources and identifying bias.

Eliz reflected on her high school education and compared it with her daughters' experience. "We researched in books, which were vetted. We had encyclopedias and dictionaries as source documents. There was a finite supply of well-sourced and vetted documents. Now all research is done online, most of which is not vetted. Kids in school have to learn how to really look at sources and decide whether or not they are trustworthy. All of us have to learn information literacy to evaluate our source documents. Are they reliable and well-vetted?"

Information literacy isn't just about understanding information; it's a series of steps, each of which requires specific skills, that better enable us to locate, evaluate, and effectively use the needed information according to the Association of College Research Libraries.

1. <u>Identify</u> the nature and extent of the information you need. *Example: Devise a search strategy about a particular health issue so you're well informed.*

2. Find the needed information effectively and efficiently.
   Example: Select the best keywords when searching online, access government website to find details about nutrition or food labeling.
3. Critically evaluate the sources you use and the information you find.
   Example: Review different sources of information, analyze the structure of arguments, research the claims made about food, scrutinize a Wikipedia article for accuracy.
4. Apply information effectively to accomplish a specific purpose.
   Example: Download an image and incorporate it into a presentation, paraphrase an expert to support your position, communicate findings about a nutrition topic.
5. Acknowledge sources of information you use.[81]
   Example: Create a works cited list while researching eating choices, attribute an image on your website or blog.

How does information literacy relate to food bullying? Being literate in handling information allows us to better identify misinformation and half-truths. This is true even when we think we know what a food claim or farming practice means so we can avoid biases. Next up I'll consider pitfalls we all must work to avoid that can derail our journey toward information literacy.

Like Socrates, assume you know little or nothing

"The only true wisdom is in knowing you know not" is a famous Socratic teaching. Unfortunately, today we take knowledge for granted. However, studies have actually shown that we often fail to understand how even everyday objects work, or to forget science that was taught to us in junior high. For example, nearly half of consumers agree that all food with DNA should be labeled, according to the 2018 MSU Food Literacy and Engagement poll. Since DNA is part of every living thing, this demonstrates that perhaps what we sometimes lack knowledge about the basic building blocks and practices associated with food.

Research on cycology in the United Kingdom demonstrated we often don't know how everyday objects work. The study used a drawing of a bicycle frame and asking respondents, which included a mix of cyclists and non-cyclists, male and female, to draw the pedals and chain. "People were found to make frequent and serious mistakes, such as believing that the chain went around the front wheel, as well as the back wheel. Errors were reduced but not eliminated for bicycle experts, for men more than women, and for people who were shown a real bicycle as they were tested. The results demonstrate that most people's conceptual understanding of this familiar, everyday object is sketchy and shallow, even for information that is frequently encountered and easily perceived," according to Rebecca Lawson in her abstract.[82]

My husband and I are cyclists; we love to ride and our local trail leads to our favorite ice cream place. This means I look at bicycles as I back out of my garage nearly every day. However, I admit that I likely wouldn't have drawn the chain and pedals in exactly the right place. Why? Because my brain is often elsewhere, or five other places when I look at our bikes, and a "conceptual understanding" of a bike isn't high on my priority list.

Isn't that true when you're making eating choices? It's not that we're ignorant about everyday objects like food, it's just that our brains are processing a lot: 100,000 chemical reactions each second and 50,000 thoughts each day. Just as we can't always correctly draw a common object, a bicycle, we don't always get it quite right about food, which we consume several times a day. It's important to remember the cycology example and keep an open mind to learning, particularly on contentious topics like GMOs, chemicals, sustainability, animal welfare, or hormones.

Beware of the Dunning-Kruger effect

While all of that is happening in our brains, there are other influences. For example, there is a psychological phenomenon known as the "Dunning-Kruger effect," where people with little expertise or ability assume they have superior expertise or ability. It's the fitness instructor making nutritional claims, the grocery store employee taking dinosaur eggs out of a mom's hand, or the mom who insists on food from a certain store be purchased for play groups. The Dunning-Kruger effect will lead a bully to embarrass others because the bully assumes his knowledge is superior.

Ryan Weeks has experienced this in Nebraska, where he farms several thousand acres of corn, soybeans, and alfalfa using irrigation. Over the last several years, Ryan has transitioned a little over half of his land into organic production so that he farms both conventionally and organically. It's an interesting combination of shared practices (cover crops) and vastly different practices (using GMO seeds and raising organic seeds). After extensive research, he has found the combination of conventional and organic management practices is best for his family, employees, and land. He has experienced taunting, shaming, and name calling from other farmers who do not agree with Ryan's choices, but those farmers may also be exhibiting the Dunning-Kruger effect. A note to my friends in agriculture: isn't it possible that there is more than one "right" way of farming and ranching?

Keep the Dunning-Kruger effect in mind when finding and evaluating information about the science, source, or system. There is a tremendous amount of wisdom, and indeed information literacy, needed to understand our everyday food choices. Most true experts will assess a variety of options or choices rather than pointing to one B.S. label or insisting on "my way or the highway."

Control for personal bias

Just as the Dunning-Kruger effect can limit our ability to take in new information and accept different practices, so can our biases. For example, I have a clear bias towards Michigan State basketball being the best basketball program in the country, and no amount of data will otherwise influence my opinion otherwise. These are known as "cognitive biases," which is just a way of saying that we create our own subjective social reality, leading us to sometimes making poor, irrational judgments in consistent patterns. It's not that we want to make these decisions. Rather, our unconscious biases can be so strong that they lead us to act in ways inconsistent with reason, values, and beliefs.

Our judgments are often inaccurate because the brain relies on cognitive biases over hard evidence, much like the emotional elephant so often controls the rational rider. Which of these biases are influencing you as you take in information and make eating decisions? I added food and farming related examples (in italics) to this *Business Insider* list showing "20 Cognitive Biases that Screw Up Your Decisions."[83]

- **Anchoring Bias:** People are over-reliant on the first piece of information they find. *In a negotiation at the farmers market, whoever makes the first offer establishes a range of reasonable possibilities.*
- **Availability heuristic:** People overestimate the importance of information available to them. *A person might argue that unlimited amounts of fat are not unhealthy because his or her grandma lived to 100 on a high fat diet.*
- **Bandwagon effect:** The probability of one person adopting a belief increases based on the number of people who hold that belief. *This is a powerful form of groupthink and why bullying spreads; consider how many times you've followed a Facebook recommendation.*

- **Blind-spot bias:** Failing to recognize your own cognitive biases is a bias itself. *It's much easier to recognize cognitive and motivational biases in others than in ourselves and judge others accordingly, particularly when food is a social statement.*

- **Choice-supportive bias:** When you choose something, you tend to feel positive about it, even if that choice has flaw. *Like how you think your homegrown brown eggs are awesome—even if they're nutritional equals with the store brand white eggs.*

- **Clustering illusion:** This is the tendency to see patterns in random events. *It's key to various fallacies, such as farmers being controlled by corporations because of lawsuits about Intellectual Property. Or do you believe scientists are unethical because of a few bad actors?*

- **Confirmation bias:** We tend to listen only to information that confirms our preconceptions. *One of the many reasons it's hard to have an intelligent conversation about climate change, different types of farming, or animal welfare. Can you have an open mind?*

- **Conservatism bias:** Where people favor prior evidence over new evidence or information that has emerged. *Your gym friend told you kale was a "superfood" five years ago, so that's more reliable than an RDN who provides data that it's just a green.*

- **Information bias:** The tendency to seek information when it does not affect action. More information is not always better; people can often make more accurate predictions with less information. *All those pretty claims on a food package aren't helping you.*

- **Ostrich effect:** The decision to ignore dangerous or negative information by burying one's head in the sand, like an ostrich. *Do you check your pantry or refrigerator when there's a food recall?*

- **Outcome bias:** Judging a decision based on the outcome, rather than how the decision was made in the moment. *Just because your child's behavior improved after you bought and served "hormone-free" meat doesn't mean that meat label was a smart decision.*

- **Overconfidence:** Some of us are too confident about our abilities, described above as the Dunning-Kruger effect. Experts are more prone to this bias than laypeople, because they are more convinced that they are right. *Try having a discussion about prices farmers receive at the farm gate compared to food prices you pay to test this.*

- **Placebo effect:** When simply believing that something will have a certain effect on you causes it to have that effect. *People given fake supplements often experience the same physiological effects as people given the real thing.*

- **Pro-innovation bias:** When a proponent of an innovation tends to overvalue its usefulness and undervalue its limitations. *Is agave really more superior than other sweeteners or does it just sound cooler?*

- **Recency:** The tendency to weigh the latest information more heavily than older data. *For example, the best definition of antibiotics dates back to 1945, but I searched for months looking for a more current one to explain antibiotics as an animal welfare tool.*

- **Salience:** Our tendency to focus on the most easily recognizable features of a person or concept. *When you think about dying, you might worry more about your food poisoning you, instead of an occurrence statistically more likely, such as a dying in a car accident.*

- **Selective perception:** Allowing our expectations to influence how we perceive the world. *You immediately* *feel better when your Arbonne representative tells you that her products will decrease intake of toxins and improve elimination of toxins, including 25 pounds of waste in your intestines. That's a lot of poop. And B.S.*

- **Stereotyping:** Expecting a group or person to have certain qualities without having real information about that person or group. It allows us to quickly identify strangers as friends or enemies, but it also builds gaps in understanding the food plate. *Do you expect farmers to wear overalls and have straw hanging out of their mouths?*

- **Survivorship bias:** An error that comes from relying only on surviving examples, causing us to misjudge a situation. *For example, we might think that farming is risk-free because we haven't heard of what happens when risks are not managed well.*

- **Zero-risk bias:** Sociologists have found that we love certainty, even if it's counterproductive. Eliminating risk completely means there is no chance of harm being caused. *Consider this: many believe that avoiding produce eliminates one's risk of chemical exposure.*

Think of the five foods you purchase most often. Which of these biases are influencing your purchasing behavior, either when eating out or grocery shopping? None of us want to be biased, but we are. Knowing which biases impact our decisions will help with information literacy.

Managing food information

Clearly the skills needed evaluate and use food information are vastly different today than even twenty years ago. Information literacy is an important skillset to help us identify and evaluate food claims. In this chapter, we have considered a process and related skill sets that can be used to create greater literacy. We have also identified common challenges in accurately evaluating information, including a number of biases and tendencies each of us need to acknowledge and overcome.

Thinking through all food-related information by understanding labels, evaluating claims, and managing information will help you overcome bullying. It may seem overwhelming, but the final section will cover how to use this food literacy to find your own solutions.

SECTION 5

Finding your own solutions

CHAPTER 18

Thinking critically to navigate the playground

Birthday cakes are a big deal in our house. Some are made from scratch; others are decorated into three-tier creations. All are designed to celebrate another year of life as a special treat. A family in Australia shares this tradition and sends leftovers to school the next day. According to LittleThings, this mom received a reprimand from her child's school after she sent a packed lunch that included a slice of the leftover, homemade chocolate cake with her kindergarten daughter the next day. "Your child has 'chocolate slice' from the Red Food category today. Please choose healthier options." This shaming note was in red ink and had a large, red, frowny face at the top.[84]

Ironically, both of the kindergartener's parents have health science degrees and emphasize healthy eating, though the frowny face food shaming note from the school may have undone some of their teaching about healthy food choices. Australia's public schools categorize different types of foods by color: green is good, yellow is O.K., and red is bad. However,

Connect with people who have firsthand expertise and critically evaluate information.

what lesson does the school send about thinking through options when they mandate food choices for children without looking at the whole picture?

Information overload

"You're drowning us in information!" My closest friends often joke about my propensity to find and digest volumes of information when there is a significant problem to be solved. Apparently, not everyone finds comfort in research. However, I'm a "fixer," and when my loved ones are facing big challenges, I turn to information about the whole picture. I once handed my friend three books in the hospital so she could properly equip herself to make decisions about her infant children. After all, how can one solve a problem without having researched all the options and possibilities?

Thankfully, I have learned that not everyone operates that way. I also have a tribe of friends who mostly tolerate my need to find as much information as possible in search of solutions. Now you know better why information literacy, a relatively new discipline, was a focus of the last chapter. Today's research looks vastly different than it did 25 years ago, thanks to social media, constant connectivity, and "fake news." Not only does research require a different approach to managing information, we have to think more critically to sort through the noise.

Increased complexity, speed, and volume of data require a higher level of critical thinking, which will be covered in this chapter. I have also found that the more contentious issues require greater levels of critical thinking to sort through the noise. When I polled my social media community, nearly every respondent said she or he was employing far more critical thinking skills today than a decade ago. Several men pointed to business reasons for increasing their critical thinking, such as the need for strategic thinking, discerning the hype, sorting through new knowledge, and marketing.

But a mom of three teens provided the most relatable example. "Parenting is not for the faint of heart. I must not allow emotion to rule my life, I have to be able to reason and look past the 'now' to a desired path of growth. Facts matter. Truth matters. We have to be able to discern fact from opinion or emotion in order to navigate all the world presents."

If you've raised a teen, you know how true this is. However, it also resonates in food. Facts matter. Truth matters. Emotions should not rule. Discerning fact from opinion will help us navigate the information overwhelm in making food and nutrition decisions for our family. Being able to quickly reason your way to a solution is the theme of this last section of *Food Bullying*.

Turn toward firsthand expertise

Stay focused on buying food that meets your family's standards and quickly cut through the claims to simplify your eating choices. Turn away from fake news and find authentic resources with firsthand expertise. As outlined below, authenticity comes from knowing the source, science, or system behind your food.

- **Know the source:** Do you have a firsthand perspective on how food is raised and why a farmer or rancher uses certain practices? They are the experts in farming and can explain why they favor certain management practices. In other words, have you visited different types of farms in the last couple of years, or do you have open access to farmers and ranchers through social media? If so, you should understand the context of animal care and environmental practices and why different food producers choose different practices.

- **Know the science:** Do you understand the science enough to evaluate health and nutrition claims on labels? Are you connected with food scientists, dietitians, and agricultural scientists who can answer questions and provide balanced, science-based recommendations? If so, you should understand scientific reasoning about how food is produced, developed, and manufactured. This will also help you understand that something can be a hazard (the potential to cause harm) without posing a serious risk (the likelihood of something causing harm). For example, an electric fence protecting cattle is a hazard to toddlers, but if it's on a ranch where toddlers are not allowed, the fence poses no risk to toddlers. Or, gluten in wheat bread is a potential hazard to a celiac but poses no risk to those not diagnosed with celiac disease.

- **Know the system:** Do you know the agricultural and food regulatory system well enough to trust and use it? Can you identify the roles of USDA, FDA, EPA, FSIS, and other regulatory bodies in keeping your food safe? Are you familiar with the requirements enforced by the system and how those affect consumers? If so, you should understand the basics of the complex system that regulates farming, food processing, manufacturing, labeling, and recalls. It may not be perfect, but it is standardized—unlike marketing claims on food.

If you are able to reach the level of self-actualization on the food buying needs hierarchy (and very few do), you will likely have a keen interest in each of above. Otherwise, consider how you can learn more about just one of these in the next month. Will you work on science, source, or system?

Discerning science from B.S.

I often hear that science is scary and that it's hard to know what is reliable. How can you tell what is sound science, whether it's about farming, food, or the regulations in place? Double X

Science offers these tips, which I find applicable in assessing what is real or not in the science surrounding food.[85]

1. Skip the headline. What is the basis of the article: original research, opinion, review of previous work?

2. What words does the author use? Link, correlation, risk, association do not mean "biological cause." In other words, just because there is an association, don't assume that is the reason for a given outcome.

3. Look at the original source of the information. Is it from a journal, a conference presentation, or a marketing campaign?

4. Remember that everyone involved in what you're reading has some return they're seeking.

5. Ask a scientist for clarification. Don't be afraid. They like to talk about science.

Double X Science also notes that Google is your friend. "Is the original source a scientific journal? At the very least, especially for original research, the abstract will be freely available. A news story based on a journal paper should provide a link to that abstract, but many, many news outlets do not do this—a huge disservice to the interested, engaged reader. At any rate, the article probably includes the name of a paper author and the journal of publication and a quick Google search on both terms, along with the subject (e.g., autism), will often locate the paper. If all you find is a news release about the paper—at outlets like ScienceDaily or PhysOrg—you are reading *marketing materials*. Period. And if there is *no mention* of publication in a journal, be very, very cautious in your interpretation of what›s being reported." [85]

Yes, that's an overwhelming amount of information! In short, carefully consider what is authentic. I have found the most authentic resources to be people with firsthand expertise.

Why critical thinking is critical

As you look at the source, science, or system, it's important to consider how you handle new stories about food. As I've continued to ask throughout *Food Bullying*, what do you do when discovering new information about food and nutrition? Do you resist it, accept it at face value and move on, analyze and debate it, or process it before formulating an opinion?

The goal of critical thinking is to try to maintain an objective position. When you think critically, you weigh all sides of an argument and evaluate its strengths and weaknesses. Critical thinking entails: actively seeking all sides of an argument, testing the soundness of the claims made, as well as testing the soundness of the evidence used to support those claims.

The following table, based on Bloom's Taxonomy,[86] gives you insight into the levels of critical thinking. I've layered in examples from the food bullying playground to show what intellectual thinking around food and farming may look like. It's important to note that different levels of critical thinking work for different situations. Don't feel like you have to hit critical evaluation on every food claim.

KNOWLEDGE

Discovering new information through observing and locating. Exhibiting memory of previously learned information.

Example: My Facebook friend posted about the hormones in meat. I know meat has hormones in it; all food has this chemical messenger of life. I talked with a farmer to learn more about how she raises animals and recall the efforts she takes to keep my meat safe.

COMPREHENSION

Demonstrating understanding of ideas and facts by organizing, translating, comparing, giving descriptors, and stating main ideas.

Example: My food does not have to be organic, which is a process managed by the USDA marketing service. In my research, I learned there are requirements to grow food organically, and it is a production choice made by some farmers. But I also know organic is not a nutritional claim.

APPLICATION

Solving problems by applying acquired knowledge, facts, techniques, and rules in a new or different way.

Example: I heard a well-known chef on TV say we should avoid gluten, but I talked to a RDN and know grain is an essential part of my diet. I like the chef, but I'm going to rely on people with firsthand expertise and continue to eat gluten since I'm not celiac. I wonder who influenced her and why?

ANALYSIS

Examining information and breaking it into parts by identifying motives or causes. Find evidence to support generalizations.

Example: This package of grapes claims non-GMO, but upon further examination, I know there are no GMO grapes. I did learn my seedless grapes are actually the outcome of breeding, and I love how convenient they are, but there's no need to worry about GMOs because they're not even an option for this product. I wonder who is trying to make money with this B.S. packaging.

SYNTHESIS

Proposing different solutions. Compiling information together in a different way or combining options into a new pattern.

Example: All of my friends are going to Restaurant X because it's "cool" and has clean, local, sustainable food. What does clean mean? How do they define local? I wondered if they're just trying to sell food, so I looked into it and found they import products from the U.K., have no definition for sustainability, and were cited for two food safety violations last year. I'm going to explain this B.S. to my friends and ask that we go to a different restaurant. I don't want to be bullied.

EVALUATION

Known as critical evaluation, this level of thinking presents and defends opinions by making judgements about information, the validity of ideas, or quality of work based on a set of criteria.

Example: These tomatoes are labeled as all-natural and chemical-free, but I know that it is B.S. because all living things are made up of chemicals. And all-natural isn't a valid label claim, either. Tomatoes are also listed on EWG's Dirty Dozen list to buy organically. Was it produced with chemicals? Likely, even if it was grown organically, because aphids love tomatoes. Besides, I know EWG's list is based on different measurements and not legitimate. Should I buy organic? I liked the way my organic tomatoes tasted last time, but they cost 40% more than regular tomatoes. Which should I choose? It seems like either is a good choice, based on my standards.

There is no one "right" answer

Critical thinking will show you that there is no one "right answer." Rather, you find the best answer for you to use in making your personal eating choices. You send that piece of leftover birthday cake in the school lunchbox, buy the spinach despite dire warning about chemicals, and ignore the carcinogen claims about ham.

Your best answer is always better than what the bullies provide. The next chapter will help you develop a simple action plan to effectively overcome bullying.

CHAPTER 19

Building a plan to overcome bullying

"When I was in college, I worked at a food co-op in Tallahassee, Florida. The store, filled with sensory experiences like the distinct smell of wheat grass being juiced, was painted with lime green borders. The co-op just made you feel good, like you were in nature or helping the earth in some way just by shopping there. Our paper grocery bags, labelled 'Co-op, stronger together,' even made you feel amazing.

"Every day at work I would hear about the 'ills' of GMOs, pesticides, chemicals, and anything non-organic from my customers and coworkers. Everyone made me think the food system was toxic, poisoning me, and harming the environment. I just assumed if everyone was so worked up about these issues, then I should be too. I had no hard evidence, it just felt right.

"I never shamed, taunted, or outwardly judged others who disagreed with me. I just thought other people didn't know or understand about the 'harms' of GMOs. I wanted to help make them aware because I care deeply

Use the six building blocks of a story as an action plan to overcome food bullying.

for the environment and farmers' quality of life. But these types of interactions were super rare because everyone I was surrounded by basically held the same beliefs as I did."

Meet Danielle Penick, a millennial RDN, who was once afraid of her food and thought she knew the one right way to eat—until a couple of years ago. I would describe her as a zealot, as she had bought into a single way of eating. She certainly had no intention of bullying, or even of being bullied, but she is a great example why we each must critically evaluate our own standards. Danielle's story will be referenced throughout this chapter as I present the different steps in developing the action plan to combat B.S.

Synthesizing your own plan

Food Bullying has given you the tools to identify the different levels of bullies, the typical bullying cycle, a hierarchy of food buying needs, tips to manage the massive flow of information, and ways to critically evaluate an issue. Now it's time to synthesize it all into a plan. I have no doubt you can do that to overcome food bullying. My six-step action plan has worked well for me in a variety of situations connecting farm and food—and I've seen others use it successfully hundreds of times. The six questions of who, what, why, where, when, and how are easy to remember; so you can tuck them away for use any time you start to doubt your eating choices. You can also get a copy of the template on the next page at https://causematters.com/foodbullying/info. Create your own plan by taking a few minutes to identify who is bullying you, their motivators, why it matters to you, where and when it's happening, and how you're going to stop it.

BUILDING YOUR OWN PLAN

1 WHO IS LIKELY TO BULLY YOU?

2 WHAT ARE THEIR MOTIVATORS?

3 WHY DOES IT MATTER TO YOU?

4 WHERE ARE YOU LIKELY TO BE BULLIED?

5 WHEN ARE YOU MOST VULNERABLE?

6 HOW CAN YOU OVERCOME THE BULLYING?

A real-world case study

Returning to Danielle's story of changing her mindset around food gives us a real-world case study to bring the action plan to life. Again, much of the food bullying likely was not intentional, but the outcomes were the same: the cycle of disconnect to distrust to fearing of food. In each of the six steps of the action plan, I've provided an example from Danielle's story and then my thoughts (in italics) on how to avoid becoming a bullying victim in your own food journey.

1. **Who?** "Many of the customers and employees at the food co-op would like to talk about how terrible irradiation, GMOs, and pesticides were and how you didn't know what your food had in it unless it was organic. I held the mindset that if it's natural, it's not bad and that anything synthetic was bad. Now I understand that it's not all or nothing; natural can be bad in some cases and synthetic can be good. The dose is the poison for everything, including water.

    "I read *Omnivores Dilemma*, which made me scared of eating anything I couldn't pronounce—I thought my food was filled with terrible things. Then, as part of my classes, I also read Marion Nestle's *Safe Food*, and it really made the biggest impression on me being very anti-GMO. She talked a lot about biotechnology, which led me to presenting a talk on avoiding GMOs for my speech class. After this, I watched "Food, Inc." It scared me and solidified my beliefs more, and I didn't see anything like this from a farmer or the ag side."

    Danielle was bullied by the groupthink of the food co-op, marketers, food influencers such as Pollan and Nestle, and documentaries. If you were to step back and write your story, who would be bullying you, intentionally or unintentionally?

2. **What?** "During the time I worked there, the labels that really scared me were the "hormone-free" and "antibiotic-free" claims because they started to make me question if everything that didn't have that label was loaded with these things. I also sought out organic labels because I was so scared of pesticides and thought that organic meant there were no pesticides in my food. Now I know organic producers use pesticides, too. I lived in constant fear of not buying food with all of the feel-good labels on it because that was reassurance I was getting 'good food'."

The labels and marketing messages mentioned called upon Danielle's needs for belonging and esteem. Which of your food buying needs are likely to be exploited by marketing labels?

3. **Why?** "I definitely had chemo-phobia. It caused me a great deal of stress to buy anything outside of the food co-op. As a college student, it was not in my budget to buy all organic health food (even with an employee discount). My mindset was to try "natural" therapies first and, if they didn't work, then I'd resort to conventional medicine like antibiotics—unless it was something more serious, like a broken bone. But that's before I realized the supplement industry isn't well regulated and how the difference between natural and conventional meds is that natural meds do become medicine once scientifically proven to be effective (and that many medicines are derived from or found directly in nature). But I was scared to eat a lot of animal products because I heard that antibiotics were in every non-organic animal product.

"My personal interests ranged from attempting to grow my own garden to learning more about cooking and foraging. I wanted to eat healthy and figured working at the store could help me eat better. But little did I know it was filled with a lot of misperceptions about nutrition and agriculture."

Danielle's emotional brain was taking her rational brain for a ride, driven by overwhelm. Are you buying food beyond your financial means or getting anxious when not shopping at your preferred store? Check in with your rational rider to be sure your emotional elephant hasn't taken over your food choices.

4. **Where?** "The best advice I can give to people is if you are following doctors, chiropractors, alternative medicine practitioners, friends, family members, nurses, or dietitians for advice on farming, agriculture, or biotechnology, I would consider also looking at what people directly involved in these areas are saying. If it's a different message than what you've heard, and it goes against everything you know to be true, try to be open minded to at least hearing this new information from the experts. Don't be so quick to dismiss it.

"Ask questions. Scientists, farmers, and experts are usually more than happy to talk to you. It's not to say that people in other specializations can't be right and aren't following the evidence in agriculture, but it's far more likely they aren't since they aren't directly involved. I can say this because I was one of those people (despite my formalized training as a dietitian). I truly thought I was right, but I wasn't, and I needed to go to different sources. I honestly thought I was following the evidence, but I wasn't. This is especially true if the people you are following are trying to sell you something with their advice. For example, it's a big red flag if they are selling you supplements, detoxes, and cleanses to detox the GMOs or pesticides or toxic chemicals."

As a dietitian, Danielle thought she knew evidence, but discovered differently when she located people with firsthand expertise. Where are you listening to those selling and missing those directly involved? Where will you find a different message about food production that goes against everything you know to be true?

5. **When?** "When I worked at the food co-op, I was at a very impressionable stage of my life as a 21-year-old living on my own for the first time. I had just started taking my core nutrition classes, and I was like a sponge. What made me most influenced by those around me was that I had wanted to work at that particular health food store for over a year and finally got hired after applying multiple times. I thought working there would help me learn more about nutrition, and the people who worked there were mostly young and were quite creative and so passionate about life. It was like a community; I wanted to be a part of it. Everyone was so interesting to me; they were musicians, poets, artists, or were nomadic—getting paid minimum wage and traveling the world. Some people lived off the grid and were into the hippie lifestyle. I was so intrigued and wanted to be a part of this community. I was still trying to figure my life out so these people I felt were a good influence to be around."

Seeking belonging during a major life change left Danielle vulnerable to the cycle of food bullying. As bullies created more disconnect and distrust, her fear of food and buying the "right" label grew. If "fear" or "right" are common in your nutrition vocabulary, you might stop to consider when you're being bullied.

6. **How?** "Changing my mind took time. Years, in fact. It wasn't one conversation, or just one person, but the result of many conversations and exposure to many resources. I

was really stubborn. After becoming an oncology dietitian, I had many patients ask about GMOs, pesticides, and other agricultural questions that I didn't always feel comfortable answering. I always wanted to know more about agriculture because it was such an unknown area to me because I was never formally trained and didn't know where to start.

"Cancer is a complex disease and often people want answers as to what caused it. Not having these answers can be frustrating and it's easy to blame certain things because you can control a lot of these variables. But you can't control the unknowns, which is what makes fear mongering messages so appealing—they're often positioned as a solution. It's easy to sell fear and tell people certain things are bad for them. And with this fear, if you give someone a simple solution, such as "buy organic," it's empowering. But with this advice, I would see people eat less produce because they couldn't afford organic or didn't have it available (myself included—I stopped eating berries and apples due to the "dirty dozen" and my fear of pesticides). And once a mind is made up, it's hard to change it with facts alone, because it's more of a feeling that causes the belief.

"Despite my beliefs, I still had questions and so did my patients, which led me to online resources. I came across the Build Up Dietitians page on Facebook and saw that the founder, RDN Leah McGrath, was always promoting really positive messages about agriculture. It made me realize almost everything I "knew" about agriculture was wrong. I was in a bit of a state of shock. It was a LOT to take in, even for someone who was seeking out this information.

"Then I started to realize that farming methods (i.e. conventional and organic) had more similarities than differences. And many farmers who grew crops and livestock conventionally, also grew crops and livestock organically. That blew my mind. It always seemed like the debate was one method vs the other. I also found The Farmer's Daughter, Farm Babe, you, SciMom, Foodie Farmer, and scientists. I was slowly changing my thinking, but still I was cautious. I was counseling cancer patients and didn't give my advice to them lightly, as RDNs are taught to be evidence-based. But this experience taught me we don't always understand science well, even if we think we are science based. It was humbling to admit that I was wrong about a lot of things.

"I married a research scientist during this time. We didn't talk about biotechnology until he was responsible for creating the world's first 'GMO' (transgenic) ant. This opened up so much dialogue. He soon realized how misinformed I was. He mentioned something along the lines of 'you know there's a scientific consensus on GMOs, right?'" It blew my mind! It was the first time that someone I actually knew and trusted said this to me. This was the nail in the coffin, so-to-speak.

"The following year, the National Academies of Science (www.nasonline.org) consensus report was published on the safety of GMOs to humans and the environment. From this point on, I felt confident about making recommendations to my patients about what to eat. We know it's worse for your health to not eat enough fruits and veggies than any potential harm that may be caused from eating the small amounts of pesticide residues found on produce.

"Now I realize that we live in one of the safest times in human history in terms of agriculture. I know that, regardless of production methods, I can feel confident in simply eating more produce and not having to worry about GMOs causing cancer or pesticide residues being harmful to me. I feel much more relaxed and less anxious. I don't have to spend an arm and a leg on expensive health foods to be healthy or worry that the agriculture industry is out to get me. I can feel confident that just simply eating more produce and whole grains, regardless of production method, is just fine. I don't worry about antibiotics or added hormones in my foods like I used to when I thought they were everywhere."

When Danielle took matters into her own hands and turned away from groupthink to find firsthand experts, she found information contrary to the fear mongering she had long bought into. How can you stand up to the bullies so you, too, can be more confident in your eating choices?

Fear is easy to sell; science isn't

When Danielle tweeted me that conversations on social media had changed her position on food and moved her from being very anti-GMO to supporting science, I knew I needed to include her story in *Food Bullying*. Through this process, she has learned to turn away from fear, which breaks the bullying cycle, as she describes below.

"Remember that fear is easy to sell, whereas the science isn't always so romantic. Data can be hard to understand, and it isn't always so dramatic as peoples' proclamations. It's also important to know that farmers are feeding themselves and their families, so it's not in their best interest to produce food that is harmful in any way—for themselves or their land. Farmers care deeply for their land and their animals. They cannot produce a good product if animals are stressed or the land is compromised.

"There are definitely pros and cons to ALL agricultural methods and there is no such thing as a panacea production method for growing food. Instead of it being a debate about what production methods are best, it would be most productive to combine best practices among all production methods. Best practices can also vary based on geography, size of the farm, and the time of year, etc. It's not always a one size fits all. If you truly believe that parts or all of agriculture are out to get you, or there is some conspiracy about agriculture, scientists, and big business being paid off to say these things, then it might be a good idea to really take a step back and re-evaluate those sources and look at the experts and science.

"Science is a process that continues to build upon its knowledge. Only until then is a consensus able to be made. I highly recommend this as it's changed my quality of life. I'm so much more relaxed now, especially now that I get to eat my berries and apples again.

"The people who were the most successful in changing my mind, however, were those who shared stories, who shared a common belief, someone who established trust and someone who explained why he or she had their public outreach. This really resonated with me. I mean we are story telling creatures and stories captivate us. People who just stated the facts and data were not nearly as effective in changing my mind."

Well said, Danielle. The stories around food need to come from those with established trust, not bullies. Danielle's path to overcoming bullying closely coincides with the six steps outlined earlier in this chapter; you can learn more about her at https://survivorstable.com. The final chapter will take a look at creating a better food story, one that includes less bullying.

CHAPTER 20

Will you be part of creating a better food story?

O ur lives are comprised of many overlapping stories, big and small. You get to choose what stories matter most in your life, but beware of how a single story can limit your thinking. Nigerian novelist Chimamanda Adichie discovered this after she was welcomed by her American college roommate with pity and expectations that Adichie would love tribal music and be unable to speak English or even use a stove. The roommate had clearly developed a stereotype of Adichie based on very limited information about African history and culture.

Adichie's Ted Talk, "The danger of a single story," is a powerful example of how we often judge others based on a single story when, in fact, she had more similarities to than differences with her college roommate. Adichie talked about how impressionable and vulnerable we are in the face of a story—and how believing a single story takes away the possibility of building human connections. She suggests we "reject a single

Know your own health, ethical, environmental, and social standards to overcome bullying and elevate the food conversation.

story" while also providing examples of single stories leading to false assumptions and even disconnect.[87]

The same is true with food. When you believe a single story, it becomes the only story—like the millennial RDN, Danielle, exemplified in the previous chapter. You stereotype food and farming based on very limited information. You reject the opportunity to understand new stories and leave yourself open to bullying.

As Adichie also wrote, "Power is the ability not just to tell the story of another person, but to make it the definitive story of that person." This final chapter will explore the power of the food story you choose to believe and how your own standards create a deeper, richer food story.

A farm girl's story grows

I grew up thinking that food had only one story—and that was the story found on the magical place known as our family farm, with pretty black and white cattle as the center of my universe. My story involved working 365 days a year with my family caring for those creatures, learning tough lessons in entrepreneurship, perseverance, compassion, and work ethic. I am thankful to be able to raise my daughter on a farm so she, too, can learn these lessons.

When I started my career, the world literally opened up while I worked internationally. I discovered the power of other cultures' stories and the vast food needs of a world outside of America. My story again diversified when I began speaking and writing to help people understand where food comes from. As I started working with people around the food plate, I realized my belief in a single story, forged during childhood, had limited my perspective and connections.

A few years later, when I became a mom, I questioned the story I had always thought to be true about food because I was so worried about making the "right" choice for my family. I found mothers with vastly different opinions than mine, books which informed me that I should only purchase one kind of food, and more 'mom judgment' than I had ever imagined. My early parenting experiences not only deepened my understanding about food, but caused me to research and determine my own standards for food. Those standards, continually evolving and adapting as I learn more about the science, source, and system of our food, have served as a solid guidepost on the chaotic playground of food marketing.

But I must say that writing *Food Bullying* has added more depth to the story than I would have imagined. Listening to a formerly homeless woman share her struggles in finding affordable food for her toddler, researching the many effects of false food labels, interviewing neuroscientists, and researching psychology brought mind-stretching dimensions. Pulling together the research for this book helped solidify the reality that we so often believe only one story about food—and become uncomfortable when encountering stories different than our own. Over time, we define our nutrition and, sometimes ourselves, by that one story. Yet, food done well is an amazing synthesis of both ingredients and stories.

Find the real stories and ingredients

The ingredients of food are likely more well-known than the real stories of how food is grown. The stories of people who care for animals in the middle of the night, the stories of a little girl who stands in her father's shadow hoping to someday take over decisions for land her great-grandpa once farmed, the stories of families who risk millions of dollars to produce food for a society who often questions them. I would ask that you consider the authentic stories of how your food is raised as a fundamental part of creating your own food story.

Like everyone, I don't have all the answers, but I do believe the experts consulted and evidence provided in this book include the ingredients of a recipe for creating a better food story to stop bullying. I realize you may have never heard of food bullying before opening this book. It's a new concept, but one of the most challenging trends in food, nutrition, and farming today. Rest assured, the food bullying playground will become larger and more chaotic if we don't address the issue head-on. Now.

If we can stop bullying, we have the opportunity to return food to its rightful place of celebration. I challenge you to find a broader, deeper story for yourself and stop the judgment around food. My hope is that the tools and ideas found in *Food Bullying* help you understand how you've been manipulated in your eating choices, the importance of stopping the B.S., and what you can do about it, beginning TODAY.

Setting your own standards

Fat-free marshmallows. Gluten-free water. Hormone-free salt. Grass-fed peaches. Vegan water. No-salt added, boneless bananas. All B.S. As discussed in the introduction of this book, the need to position one food as superior to another lies at the heart of food bullying. These label claims fly in the face of my food standards (and drive me crazy); so I turn away from food with these types of claims. It's an example of how overcoming bullying begins with knowing your own food standards and using them as guideposts on the chaotic playground.

Below are the four standards I've referenced throughout this book, with a key question associated with each standard for you to consider. I've provided my own beliefs for each standard as an example; use them, if you choose, as fodder in developing your own standards.

Health standard

- *Example: I do not believe food is medicine, but do contend that care of our health must be proactive. Understanding the science of nutrition, eating a balanced diet, and exercising are key to my family's health. I believe food should be experienced with joy, not guilt, and should also be a central part of our family traditions (especially chocolate and ice cream). Further, I believe we have a responsibility to ensure the health of global citizens through adequate nourishment.*

- What health priorities influence your food choices?

_____

_____

_____

_____

Ethical standard

- *Example: I believe that animals and the earth deserve honorable care, but I do not value either above humans. I believe ethics in food should include taking responsibility for a safe product, seeking truth from experts and identifying more honest marketing. I trust the system in place to protect our food and I believe that improvements come from science. And I take ethical issue with those who try to bully others at any level, particularly those who slander farmers and ranchers in order to advance their narrow, self-serving agendas.*

- What ethical principles influence your food choices?

_____

_____

_____

_____

Environmental standard

- *I believe sustainability is multi-faceted. I believe soil is a farm's greatest asset, in both modern and traditional farming practices that protect our environment. I also believe animals are natural recyclers, efficiency in production matters and that true sustainability includes long-term economic viability for businesses. I take personal responsibility for my environmental impact and hope to improve that for future generations through science. However, I will continue to question the 'quick-fix' campaigns so often proposed.*

- What environmental concerns influence your food choices?

_____

_____

_____

_____

Social Standard

- *I deeply believe in personal choice. I believe in making decisions for the benefit of my family and the good of society, but I will not participate in groupthink. I seek and value my community's input, but I do not rely on it to make decisions for my family or about our social well-being. I do not believe a marketing claim equates to social responsibility for a company, but that actions speak louder. I hold myself to the same accountability. I also believe that food and drink are central to our social gatherings and are integral to celebrating family and friends.*

- What social connections influence your food choices?

_____

_____

_____

_____

Knowing and trusting your own health, ethical, environmental, and social standards will help you stand up to the bullies and take fear out of the food equation. What do you believe about the food you put into your body? You don't need to have a long mission statement around food. Just know where you stand and don't allow fear mongering and unethical marketing to sway you. Take a few minutes to come up with your general beliefs for each standard so you have guideposts. They don't have to be eloquently written, but getting them on paper will help you solidify your own food standards.

Lose the bad food feelings

Once you know your standards and what you believe to be true about food, remember this from author Brené Brown: "Shame is the most powerful, master emotion. It's the fear that we're not good enough." Food should never be about shame. Food should never be a statement about whether you're good enough. And others should never be shaming you about food. Really.

Nor should you be shaming yourself about eating choices and that one negative story we tend to repeat over and over. Is it what you were told as a kid? Or a hurtful statement that was made to you a decade ago? Is it the definitive story of your nutrition choices?

"I'm fat and need to be on a diet. I don't deserve to eat tasty food."

"X will give me cancer."

"I can't cook, so buying fresh food is a waste of money."

"My children will be damaged if I don't feed them Y."

"I'm unhealthy, so it doesn't matter if I eat unhealthy food."

"I'm not going to buy fresh produce because it rots."

"My kids are only happy when I buy Z."

"I'm too busy to cook healthy food."

The point is, don't overlook the possibility that you may be bullying yourself over that one-line-story that was told to you a decade (or more) ago. I know I have been guilty of self-bullying. If it's words you wouldn't tolerate others saying, why are you saying them to yourself?

Use WHY? as a fear filter

It's time to lose the bad feelings about food and walk away from the story shaming you about food. Food is a basic necessity, not a political statement. Unfortunately, disconnect and distrust have created a food playground filled with fairytales. Asking WHY can help you filter a lot of fear around food.

Keep your anti-bullying "WHY? fear filter" on as you have the tough conversations about eating choices. Here are seven simple ways to break the bullying cycle, with some examples for each:

- **Listen for stories:** Ask people to share stories about their lives, interests, family, etc. Identify what's important to them and why so you can develop a personal connection.
  Example: Why would a grocery store employee take dinosaur eggs out of a shopper's hand? Concerns for safety and fear create knee-jerk reactions.

- **Examine the intention:** Differentiate between the person's intent and the impact on you.
  Example: Why would Chipotle produce a video to make people question how food is produced? Likely because they want to sell food, branded with their claims.

- **Know when you don't know:** Consider context instead of drama and sensationalized misinformation. If you don't know what you don't you know, ask someone with firsthand experience. Always ask why.
  Example: Why do farmers dehorn and trim tails on animals? It may appear incredibly cruel, but it is crueler to allow animals to injure each other or the people working with the animals.

- **Check your biases and motivators:** Pay attention to your own reactions and keep the emotional brain in check. Where does the food claim fall on the hierarchy?
  Example: Why would a superfood, weenie water, or special supplement make me feel better and look younger? Consider if any biases are clouding your judgement.

- **Change the interaction:** Find common ground; seek comic relief when you need to break the tension. Try to take the conversation off of emotional center, if possible.

Remember that's it's O.K. to disagree—and that others are watching.

Example: Why would one farmer who chooses to farm conventionally want to talk to one who farms organically? Talking regularly helps them find common practice, learn new ideas—and "shoot the breeze" to laugh a little while blowing off steam about the pressures of farming.

- **Call out a food bully:** Use the food buying needs hierarchy to identify moments of bullying. Help others to do the same. Turn away from food packages with bullying labels.

  Example: Why are they removing food choices? A school system makes noise about being more environmentally friendly by proposing a 'Meatless Monday' policy while failing to provide a variety of fresh fruits and vegetables every day—an example of putting misinformed 'groupthink' before nutrition. Work with other parents to find the environmental and nutritional truth for the proposed policy, send emails to the school board and administrators, and make a point to attend meetings to express your concerns about nutritional choices being available. Speak out when food bullying is used to create regulations that make food more expensive.

- **Find and tell your own story.** It matters, more than you know. We need a playground filled with truth that supports choice in eating, not the chaos of food bullying.

  Example: Why does your story matter? Stories built on strong health, ethical, environmental, and social standards keep bullies at bay. Consider Danielle, once a zealot terrified of food while searching for belonging, who eventually finds her way through the various food buying needs to self-actualization. She no longer associates food with fear and, as a RDN, helps others do the same.

Pick which of these ideas apply to you and your situation. Use them to create a better food story, always after you've asked WHY? After all, if we could have a civilized food conversation, perhaps we could also find a way to create more civility in our politics, personal lives, and professional communications. Are you in? This is your chance to engage.

Filling the space with a better story

Stories can lead people down the wrong path and create a powerful division around food, as demonstrated time and time again throughout these pages. Stories can also unite people and return food to a place of celebration and tradition. It is time we find a better food story.

However, if you take away one story about food misinformation, research shows you have to fill it with another story. "When people hear misinformation, they build a mental model, with the myth providing an explanation. When the myth is debunked, a gap is left in their mental model. To deal with this dilemma, people prefer an incorrect model over an incomplete model. In the absence of a better explanation, they opt for the wrong explanation."[88] It's important to note that explicit warnings reduce but do not eliminate the continued influence of misinformation.

In other words, your brain will revert to the false information if you leave a blank space where that story once existed. The only way to solve this problem, in relation to food bullying, is to be really clear about your own food story. Clarify your story by identifying your own standards, using WHY? to filter fear and giving yourself permission to mentally stand up to 200,000+ bullying claims.

Here is an experiment for the next time you buy food. Let's call it the **"No B.S. Food Challenge"** to help you fill the space with your own story.

- How easy is it to find food without B.S. labels?

- Can you fill your plate with choices made without bullying influences?
- Share a #NoBSFood photo on Instagram, Facebook Live, or a tweet to help others and show me how you're putting *Food Bullying* to work.

I believe in choice. And civil conversation.

I believe that a cornerstone of any food story is choice. Eating is a deeply personal choice, as is farming. You may choose to eat or farm completely differently than me. But does that mean we cannot engage in civil conversation? I hope not.

It's time to change the dynamics of how we handle disagreement and elevate the conversation around food. That starts with you. The next time you're involved in a discussion about eating choices, use these tools to identify the other person's behavior, but also check your own. It's difficult, but essential, if we want to have civil discourse.

"We cannot solve our problems with the same think we used when we created them," said Albert Einstein. Little did he know how true those words would be in the 21st century. Isn't it time that we use a different "think" to recognize food bullying for what it is and stop buying B.S.? Today is a great time for you to begin creating a better food story!

FINAL THOUGHTS

Standing up for what is right

The food playground is bigger than I realized when I began writing *Food Bullying*. 50,000 words later, I have learned that the chaos reaches well beyond than the typical players arguing about food and topics du jour. The playground of food bullying includes more psychological maneuvering than most of us understand. Throw on some neuroscience, and the playground becomes a virtual cauldron of heated debate.

Our brain's response to information about food is fascinating and in the earliest stages of research. I am excited to look further into the intersection of our brain behavior and the various influences on that behavior. Given the $5.75 trillion business of food, I am certain this neuroscience information will be exploited as a marketing tool that will lead to even more bullying. The anecdote to bullying is standing up for what is right.

Today's contentious food environment involves a lot of manipulation. I don't pretend to have all the answers, but I do believe in standing up for what is right. That is the truth in food. I know if readers stand for truth and employ the tools outlined in this book, we can start breaking the bullying cycle. Keep sharing your stories and #NoBSfood images with me (@mpaynspeaker) about how you are able to overcome bullies and Bull Speak. As more people are aware of food bullying, the playground will become less chaotic and healthier for all of us.

I happen to believe food—and the choices we make—should be simpler. Don't you? It's time to stand up for what is right.

NOTES

Chapter 1

1.   Hauf, Lisa. 2018. *On Your Table.* August 24. Accessed November 6, 2018. https://ndfb.org/on-your-table/on-your-table-blog/dinosaur-eggs-and-roundup/.

Chapter 2

2.   *Pacer's National Bullying Prevention Center.* n.d. Accessed December 9, 2018. https://www.pacer.org/bullying/resources/parents/definition-impact-roles.asp.

3.   Piper, Kelsey. 2019. *Vox.* January 29. Accessed October 19, 2018. https://www.vox.com/future-perfect/2018/10/31/18026418/vegan-vegetarian-animal-welfare-corporate-advocacy.

4.   MacDonald, PhD, Ruth. 2018. *Genetic Literacy Project.* August 8. Accessed December 6, 2018. https://geneticliteracyproject.org/2018/08/08/nutritionist-reflects-sad-state-health-education-gmos-farming-schools-universities/?mc_cid=7804fe6030&mc_eid=48142ccabe.

5.   Sagan, Aleksandra. 2019. *www.meatbusiness.ca.* February 7. Accessed February 10, 2019. http://www.meatbusiness.ca/2018/12/05/average-family-to-pay-400-more-for-groceries-next-year/.

6.   Comen, Evan, Frohlich, Thomas. 2018. *USA Today. com.* July 16. Accessed January 9, 2019. https://www.usatoday.com/story/money/personalfinance/2018/07/16/what-groceries-driving-up-food-bill-look-

top-20/776106002/.

Chapter 3

7.   *The Statistics Portal.* n.d. Accessed February 11, 2019.
      https://www.statista.com/topics/1660/food-retail/.

Chapter 4

8.   Brown, Dalvin. 2018. *USA Today.* June 21. Accessed
      October 26, 2018. https://www.usatoday.com/story/
      money/2018/06/21/hot-dog-water-sold-38-bottle-cana-
      dian-festival/721055002/.
9.   Steussy, Lauren. 2018. *New York Post.* Octo-
      ber 23. Acessed October 29, 2018. https://nypost.
      com/2018/10/23/your-mealprep-obsession-could-sig-
      nal-an-eating-disorder/.
10.   Rumsey, Alissa. 2018. *U.S. News.* September 4. Ac-
      cessed October 6, 2018. https://health.usnews.com/
      health-news/blogs/eat-run/articles/2018-09-04/enjoy-
      your-food-its-good-for-your-health.
11.   Austrew, Ashley. 2017. *Café Mom.* November 7. Ac-
      cessed December 4, 2018. https://thestir.cafemom.com/
      parenting_news/208510/mom_viral_post_lunch_sham-
      ing.

Chapter 5

12.   Stanley, T.L. 2018. *Adweek.* November 28. Ac-
      cessed December 9, 2018. https://www.adweek.com/
      brand-marketing/payless-opened-a-fake-luxury-store-
      palessi-to-see-how-much-people-would-pay-for-20-
      shoes/.
13.   IFIC. 2019. *Food Insight.* January. Accessed March
      4, 2019. https://foodinsight.org/wp-content/up-
      loads/2019/01/IFIC-FDN-AHA-Report.pdf.
14.   2018. *Michigan State University.* October 10. Accessed
      October 22, 2018. https://www.canr.msu.edu/news/msu-

food-literacy-and-engagement-poll-wave-iii.

15. Jones, Julie. 2012. *Wheat Belly—An Analysis of Selected Statements and Basic Thesis from the Book.* 4. Vol. 57. https://aaccipublications.aaccnet.org/doi/pdf/10.1094/CFW-57-4-0177.

16. 2010. *U.S. Food and Drug Administration.* April. Accessed February 26, 2019. https://www.fda.gov/Food/IngredientsPackagingLabeling/FoodAdditivesIngredients/ucm094211.htm#how.

17. *U.S. Department of Agriculture.* n.d. Accessed January 9, 2019. https://www.ams.usda.gov/rules-regulations/be/bioengineered-foods-list.

18. Campbell, Andrew. 2018. *Real Agriculture.* April 5. Accessed November 4, 2018. https://www.realagriculture.com/2018/04/cfia-now-says-non-gmo-project-verified-doesnt-mean-non-gmo/.

Chapter 6

19. Loy, Dan. 2011. *Iowa Beef Center.* March. Accessed December 12, 2018. http://www.iowabeefcenter.org/information/IBC48.pdf.

20. Basarab, John, et al. 2012. *U.S. National Library of Medicine National Institutes of Health.* April 16. Accessed January 9, 2019. https://www.ncbi.nlm.nih.gov/pmc/articles/PMC4494322/.

21. Kaplowitz, Paul. 2006. *Research Gate.* November. Accessed March 4, 2019. https://www.researchgate.net/publication/6856460_Pubertal_development_in_girls_Secular_trends.

22. Katiraee, Layla. 2018. *Sci Moms.* November 1. Accessed December 9, 2018. https://scimoms.com/2018/11/01/hormones_in_food/.

Chapter 7

23. Henderson, Greg. 2018. *AgWeb.* October 31. Accessed November 9, 2018. https://www.agweb.com/article/size-doesnt-matter-for-animal-welfare/.

24. Balmford, Andrew, et al. 2018. *Nature Sustainability.* September 14. Accessed January 9, 2019. https://www.nature.com/articles/s41893-018-0138-5.

25. Bovay, John, Ferrier, Peyton, Zhen, Chen. 2018. *U.S. Department of Agriculture.* August. Accessed March 20, 2019. https://www.ers.usda.gov/webdocs/publications/89749/eib-195.pdf?v=43319.

Chapter 8

26. Mitloehner, Frank. 2018. *Business Insider.* December 25. Accessed January 9, 2019. https://www.businessinsider.com/giving-up-meat-wont-save-planet-2018-10.

27. 2016. *EPA.* Accessed March 20, 2019. https://www.epa.gov/ghgemissions/overview-greenhouse-gases.

28. Mottet, Anne, Steinfeld, Henning. 2018. *Thomson Reuters Foundation News.* September 18. Accessed March 27, 2019. http://news.trust.org/item/20180918083629-d2wf0.

Chapter 9

29. Houlihan, Jane. n.d. *Activist Facts.* Accessed March 27, 2019. https://www.activistfacts.com/?s=ewg+-says+that+the+group+overstates.

30. Huang, Yancui, Edirisinghe, Indika, Burton-Freeman, Britt. 2016. *Nutrition Today Online.* September/October. Accessed January, 13 2019. https://journals.lww.com/nutritiontodayonline/Fulltext/2016/09000/Low_Income_Shoppers_and_Fruit_and_Vegetables__What.6.aspx.

31. 2016. *Center for Disease Control and Prevention.* February 1. Accessed January 27, 2019. https://www.cdc.gov/ecoli/2015/o26-11-15/index.html.

32. Redman, Russell. 2018. *Supermarket News.* September 6. Accessed January 27, 2019. https://www.supermarketnews.com/retail-financial/whole-foods-store-employees-look-unionize.

Chapter 10

33. Srivastav, Ajay. 2018. *The Hindu Business Line.* April 17. Accessed February 12, 2019. https://www.thehindubusinessline.com/opinion/columns/ajay-srivastav/how-india-can-become-a-5-trillion-economy/article23562940.ece.

34. *The Statistics Portal.* n.d. Accessed February 12, 2019. https://www.statista.com/topics/1660/food-retail/.

35. Danziger, Pamela. 2018. *Forbes.* December 30. Accessed February 12, 2019. https://www.forbes.com/sites/pamdanziger/2018/12/30/will-dollar-stores-be-the-end-of-local-american-retail-ilsr-seems-to-think-so/#3304331d6194.

36. 2018. *Food and Agriculture Organization.* Accessed February 26, 2019. http://www.fao.org/state-of-food-security-nutrition/en/.

37. Cunnane, Caroline. 2018. *Dirt to Dinner.* June 7. Accessed February 12, 2019. https://www.dirt-to-dinner.com/dear-juice-press.

38. Shropshire, Corilyn. 2018. *Washington Post.* July 15. Accessed February 12, 2019. https://www.washingtonpost.com/national/health-science/what-you-need-to-know-about-food-recalls/2018/07/13/4fbd294e-74b8-11e8-805c-4b67019fcfe4_story.html.

39. Maze, Jonathan. 2018. *Restaurant Business Online.* January 3. Accessed January 12, 2019. https://www.

restaurantbusinessonline.com/financing/panera-breads-sales-thrive-thanks-digital.
40. Fielding-Singh, Priya. 2018. *Los Angeles Times.* February 7. Accessed February 12, 2019. https://www.latimes.com/opinion/op-ed/la-oe-singh-food-deserts-nutritional-disparities-20180207-story.html.
41. Baker, Sinéad. 2018. *Business Insider.* July 26. Accessed February 10, 2019. https://www.businessinsider.com/gwyneth-paltrow-didnt-want-goop-articles-fact-checked-monetize-eyeballs-2018-7.

Chapter 11
42. Viswanathan, Radhika. 2018. *Vox.* December 21. Accessed February 1, 2019. https://www.vox.com/2018/6/25/17488336/plastic-straw-ban-ocean-pollution.
43. Wellman, Barry. 2011. *The British Journal of Psychology.* August 8. Accessed February 12, 2019. http://groups.chass.utoronto.ca/netlab/wp-content/uploads/2012/05/Is-Dunbars-Number-Up.pdf.
44. Carroll, Conn. 2012. *Washington Examiner.* January 9. Accessed February 13, 2019. https://www.washingtonexaminer.com/critics-question-spending-by-humane-society-of-the-united-states.
45. Markman, Ph.D., Art. 2010. *Psychology Today.* August 31. Accessed February 9, 2019. https://www.psychologytoday.com/us/blog/ulterior-motives/201008/what-does-advertising-do.
46. 2018. *EurekAlert!.* December 3. Accessed February 12, 2019. https://www.eurekalert.org/pub_releases/2018-12/sfra-tic111918.php.
47. Taylor, Kate. 2018. *Business Insider.* October 8. Accessed February 22, 2019. https://www.businessinsider.com/lacroix-responds-lawsuit-natural-ingredients-2018-10.

48. Park, Michael. 2014. *Bon Appetit.* October 30. Accessed December 12, 2018. https://www.bonappetit.com/test-kitchen/how-to/article/supermarket-psychology.

Chapter 12

49. Lewandowsky, Stephan, et al. 2012. *Association for Psychological Science.* Accessed March 5, 2019. https://dornsife.usc.edu/assets/sites/780/docs/12_pspi_lewandowsky_et_al_misinformation.pdf.
50. Koger, Chris. 2018. *Ag Web.* September 3. Accessed January 22, 2019. https://www.agweb.com/article/report-new-california-regulations-pass-203-million-to-citrus-growers/.
51. Kaiser, Harry. 2016. *Cornell University.* May. Accessed February 22, 2019. http://publications.dyson.cornell.edu/docs/smartMarketing/pdfs/SmrtMkgMay2016.pdf.
52. Davis, Tyler, LaCour, Mark, Beyer, Erin, Miller, Markus. 2019. *bioRxiv. The Reprint Server for Biology.* April 1. Accessed April 2, 2019. https://www.biorxiv.org/content/10.1101/595314v1.
53. Seth, Anil. 2017. *30-Second Brain.* New York, NY: Metro Books.
54. Cantor Ph.D, Joanne. 2011. *Psychology Today.* February 27. Accessed February 22, 2019. https://www.psychologytoday.com/us/blog/conquering-cyber-overload/201102/flooding-your-brain-s-engine-how-you-can-have-too-much-good.
55. Ellis, Esther. 2018. *Food & Nutrition.* September 20. Accessed December 20, 2018. https://foodandnutrition.org/from-the-magazine/at-the-supermarket-whats-trending/.
56. Harris, PhD, MBA, Jennifer. 2019. *Rudd Report.* January. Accessed February 28, 2019. http://uconnruddcen-

ter.org/files/Pdfs/TargetedMarketingReport2019.pdf.

Chapter 13

57. Seth, Anil. 2017. *30-Second Brain.* New York, NY: Metro Books.
58. Prodan, Diana. 2018. *Skyword.* November 2. Accessed February 26, 2019. https://www.skyword.com/content-standard/marketing/the-psychology-of-social-sharing-what-makes-people-engage-with-your-social-media-content/.
59. Ryan, PhD, Cami. 2016. *Cami Ryan, PhD.* April 21. Accessed February 19, 2019. https://camiryan.com/2016/04/21/ready-set-shame-the-shame-game-in-modern-advertising-and-modern-life/.
60. Yan, Holly. 2018. *CNN.* August 11. Accessed March 20, 2019. https://www.cnn.com/2018/08/10/health/monsanto-johnson-trial-verdict/index.html.
61. ACSH Staff. 2018. *American Council on Science and Health.* October 9. Accessed October 22, 2018. https://www.acsh.org/news/2018/10/09/if-you-accept-science-you-accept-roundup-does-not-cause-cancer-13490.
62. Lanford, LDN, Julie. 2015. *Cancer Dietitian.* August 12. Accessed February 16, 2019. https://www.cancerdietitian.com/wordpress/2015/08/why-you-should-stop-saying-sugar-feeds-cancer.html.

Chapter 14

63. Tapp, W.N., et al. 2017. *ScienceDirect.* April. Accessed March 4, 2019. https://www.sciencedirect.com/science/article/abs/pii/S0309174016306234.
64. Davis, Tyler, LaCour, Mark, Beyer, Erin, Miller, Markus. 2019. *bioRxiv. The Reprint Server for Biology.* April 1. Accessed April 2, 2019. https://www.biorxiv.org/content/10.1101/595314v1.
65. Barth, F. Diane. 2017. *Psychology Today.* February 7.

Accessed March 4, 2019. https://www.psychologyto-day.com/us/blog/the-couch/201702/6-smarter-ways-deal-bully.

66. 2019. *Food Insight.* January 24. Accessed March 4, 2019. https://foodinsight.org/food-labeling/.

Chapter 15

67. Mikkelson, David. 2018. *Snopes.* August 10. Accessed December 5, 2018. https://www.snopes.com/fact-check/bacon-package-cooking-instructions/.

68. 2018. *Michigan State University.* October 10. Accessed March 5, 2019. https://www.canr.msu.edu/news/msu-food-literacy-and-engagement-poll-wave-iii.

69. *U.S. Food and Drug Administration.* n.d. Accessed March 12, 2019. https://www.fda.gov/downloads/Food/GuidanceRegulation/GuidanceDocumentsRegulatoryInformation/UCM265446.pdf.

70. *Healthy Living.* n.d. Accessed March 12, 2019. https://www.heart.org/en/healthy-living/company-collaboration/heart-check-certification/heart-check-in-the-grocery-store/heart-check-food-certification-program-nutrition-requirements.

71. *Oldways Whole Grains Council.* n.d. Accessed March 12, 2019. https://wholegrainscouncil.org/whole-grain-stamp.

Chapter 16

72. D'Entremont, Yvette. 2016. *Cosmopolitan.* January 11. Accessed March 5, 2019. https://www.cosmopolitan.com/health-fitness/news/a51998/all-of-the-reasons-why-tom-and-giseles-diet-is-actually-the-worst-revealed.

73. 2010. *U.S. Food and Drug Administration.* March 3. Accessed March 5, 2019. http://wayback.archive-it.org/7993/20170406011336/https://www.fda.gov/Food/

IngredientsPackagingLabeling/LabelingNutrition/ucm202733.htm.

74. *U.S. Food and Drug Administration.* n.d. Accessed March 5, 2019. https://www.fda.gov/Food/Guidance-Regulation/GuidanceDocumentsRegulatoryInformation/LabelingNutrition/ucm217762.htm.

75. 2016. *U.S. Food and Drug Administration.* May 20. Accessed March 1, 2019. https://www.fda.gov/food/guidanceregulation/guidancedocumentsregulatoryinformation/labelingnutrition/ucm385663.htm.

76. *U.S. Food and Drug Administration.* n.d. Accessed March 12, 2019. https://www.fda.gov/Food/IngredientsPackagingLabeling/FoodAllergens/ucm079311.htm.

77. Neff, Roni, et al. 2019. *Science Direct.* February 12. Accessed March 5, 2019. https://www.sciencedirect.com/science/article/pii/S0956053X19300194?via%3Dihub.

78. *U.S. Department of Agriculture.* n.d. Accessed March 5, 2019. https://www.fsis.usda.gov/wps/portal/fsis/topics/food-safety-education/get-answers/food-safety-factsheets/food-labeling/food-product-dating/food-product-dating.

79. *U.S. Department of Agriculture.* n.d. Accessed March 12, 2019. https://www.fsis.usda.gov/wps/portal/fsis/topics/food-safety-education/get-answers/food-safety-factsheets/safe-food-handling/basics-for-handling-food-safely/ct_index.

Chapter 17

80. Lewandowsky, Stephan, et al. 2012. *Association for Psychological Science.* Accessed December 15, 2019. http://www.emc-lab.org/uploads/1/1/3/6/113627673/lewandowskyecker.2012.pspi.pdf.

81. Gupta, Priyanka. n.d. *Ed Tech Review*. Accessed March 11, 2019. http://edtechreview.in/trends-insights/insights/2783-information-literacy-skills.

82. Lawson, Rebecca. 2006. *Springer Link*. December. Accessed March 10, 2019. https://link.springer.com/article/10.3758/BF03195929.

83. Lebowitz, Shana, Lee, Samantha. 2015. *Business Insider*. August 25. Accessed March 12, 2019. https://www.businessinsider.com/cognitive-biases-that-affect-decisions-2015-8.

Chapter 18

84. Endicott, Rebecca. n.d. *Little Things*. Accessed April 3, 2019. https://www.littlethings.com/chocolate-cake-angry-note.

85. 2012. *Double X Science*. April 27. Accessed March 11, 2019. http://www.doublexscience.com/2012/04/science-health-medical-news-freaking.html.

86. *Open Learn*. n.d. Accessed March 1, 2019. https://www.open.edu/openlearn/ocw/mod/oucontent/view.php?id=51387&section=4.

Chapter 20

87. Adichie, Chimamanda. 2009. *Ted Talk*. July. Accessed October 11, 2018. https://www.ted.com/talks/chimamanda_adichie_the_danger_of_a_single_story.

88. Ecker, Ullrich, Lewandowsky, Stephan, Tang, DT. 2010. *U.S. National Library of Medicine National Institutes of Health*. December. Accessed March 11, 2019. https://www.ncbi.nlm.nih.gov/pubmed/21156872.

GRATITUDE

"Thank you" is one the most powerful phrases in the English language. My husband, Erik, has encouraged me from the moment I decided to write *Food Bullying* and continued that through the writing process with shoulder massages, feeding our cattle and picking up home front pieces I dropped. The same "thank you" goes to Elle, my office manager, for the citations, formatting, and cheering me on. I appreciate both of you more than you know.

Kirk, I never thought you'd be editing my book after you were my go-to advisor in college, but it has been a privilege to have your "red pen" honing *Food Bullying*. Special thanks to Eliz for the countless Facetime calls debating health, bias and farming; to Jennie, who inspired me to write this book; Cami for offering mind boggling research; and to Ellen, an unwavering friend who feeds me food questions and fashion ideas.

Thank you to the neuroscientists, farmers, psychologists, dietitians, ranchers, veterinarians and health professionals who so willingly shared their expertise and research. Nearly 50 people served as an 'advisory community' throughout the development of this book—I appreciated the invaluable guidance from all sides of the plate. There are too many others who helped to recognize each individually, but the stories about food bullying I received from friends and strangers unquestionably inspired this book, particularly Danielle's powerful story of change.

Audiences from across the food, agriculture and health arenas offered fodder over nearly 20 years of my speaking about these issues. The same can be said of my online communities—sometimes just a question, idea, or simple comment helped guide the book. Thanks for the AHA moments!

"A life without cause is a life without effect," a quote above my desk, serves as a daily reminder of the cause of returning food to its rightful place of celebration. Working for a cause is a choice and commitment I hope my daughter and stepdaughters can learn from; may *Food Bullying* remind you to always stand up for what you believe in.

ABOUT THE AUTHOR

Michele Payn, an international, award-winning author, brings clarity and common sense to the emotional food conversation. Known as one of North America's leading voices in connecting farm and food, Michele helps you simplify safe food choices.

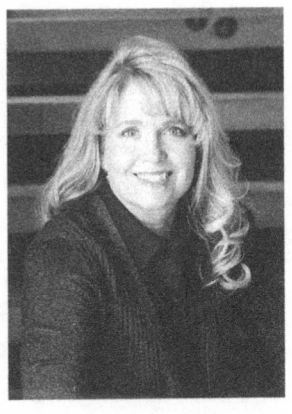

She is an in-demand media resource whose work has appeared in *USA Today*, NPR, CNN, Food Insight, *Food & Nutrition Magazine*, *Grist* and others. Michele has spoken before hundreds of groups including dietetic Associations, universities, Aetna, Michigan Vegetable Growers, Farm Credit Council and farm bureaus in 40+ states—helping thousands of people around the world connect farm and food. In addition to a lifetime on the farm, Michele has:

- Authored two books: *Food Truths from Farm to Table*, selected as a bronze medal recipient from among 5,500 books entered in the Independent Publishers Book Awards (IPPY), the world's largest book contest and *No More Food Fights!*
- Earned the Certified Speaking Professional designation awarded to less than eight percent of professional speakers globally, after speaking to 500+ groups.

- Founded AgChat and FoodChat, virtual communities connecting more than 20,000 farmers, dietitians, chefs, foodies, agribusinesses and ranchers from 20 countries.
- Received B.S. degrees in Agricultural Communications and Animal Science from Michigan State University, where the story of her impact has been featured in a Spartan Saga alumni profile.
- Worked with farmers in 25 countries, raised millions of dollars for education and built a successful business, Cause Matters Corp.

Michele Payn is a mom who is tired of food bullying. She enjoys working on her small farm in Indiana with her "city slicker" husband and cow-loving daughter, as well as cooking, making memories with friends, coaching 4-H & FFA members, traveling and cheering on the Michigan State Spartans.

Connect with Michele

Has *Food Bullying* changed the way you make eating choices? Do you have food bullying stories you'd like to share? Are questions popping up as you buy food with a personal plan and heightened awareness? Michele would love to hear from you at book@causematters.com.

Want to bring her *Food Bullying* expertise to your people? Discover for yourself why audiences rave about Michele's high energy, interactive speaking programs and unique ability to engage everyone around the food table. Learn more at www.causematters. com or connect with @mpaynspeaker across social media.

- Twitter: http://www.twitter.com/mpaynspeaker
- Facebook: http://facebook.com/causematters
- Instagram: http://www.instagram.com/mpaynspeaker
- Linkedin: www.linkedin.com/in/mpaynspeaker

Thanks for helping clean up the chaos and keeping bullies off the food playground.

OTHER BOOKS BY MICHELE PAYN

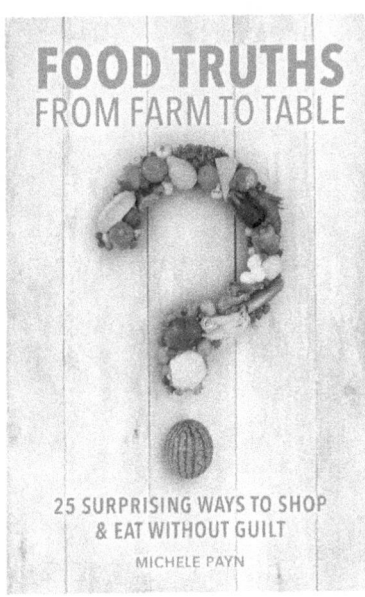

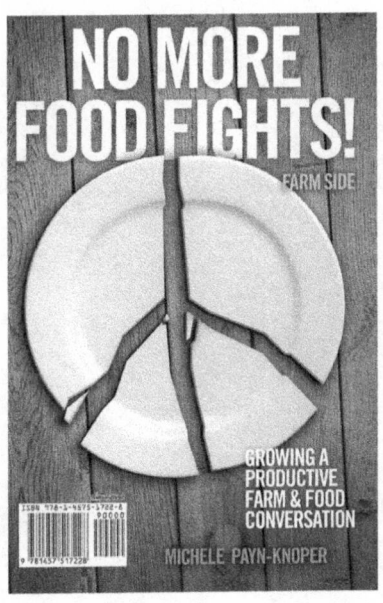